Community Palliative Care

Community Palliative Care
The Role of the Clinical Nurse Specialist

Alexandra M. Aitken

MSc in Primary Care, BA in Community Health Studies,
Registered Nurse, Registered Midwife and Specialist
Practitioner – District Nursing

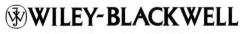

A John Wiley & Sons, Ltd., Publication

This edition first published 2009
© 2009 by Alexandra M. Aitken

Blackwell Publishing was acquired by John Wiley & Sons in February 2007. Blackwell's publishing programme has been merged with Wiley's global Scientific, Technical, and Medical business to form Wiley-Blackwell.

Registered office
John Wiley & Sons Ltd, The Atrium, Southern Gate, Chichester, West Sussex, PO19 8SQ, United Kingdom

Editorial offices
9600 Garsington Road, Oxford, OX4 2DQ, United Kingdom
350 Main Street, Malden, MA 02148-5020, USA

For details of our global editorial offices, for customer services and for information about how to apply for permission to reuse the copyright material in this book please see our website at www.wiley.com/wiley-blackwell.

The right of the author to be identified as the author of this work has been asserted in accordance with the Copyright, Designs and Patents Act 1988.

Library of Congress Cataloging-in-Publication Data
Aitken, Alexandra M.
Community palliative care : the role of the clinical nurse specialist / Alexandra M. Aitken.
    p. ; cm.
  Includes bibliographical references and index.
  ISBN 978-1-4051-8076-4 (pbk. : alk. paper) 1. Palliative treatment. 2. Terminal care.
3. Community health nursing . 4. Hospice nurses. I. Title.
  [DNLM: 1. Palliative Care–Great Britain. 2. Community Health Nursing–Great Britain. 3. Nurse's Role–Great Britain. WY 152 A311c 2009]

  RT87.T45.A38 2009
  616′.029—dc22

                                                          2008034862

A catalogue record for this book is available from the British Library.

Set in 10/13 pt Palatino by Newgen Imaging Systems Pvt Ltd, Chennai
Printed in Malaysia by KHL Printing Co Sdn Bhd
1   2009

Contents

Introduction

Community palliative care clinical nurse specialists (commonly known as Macmillan nurses) play an important role in specialist palliative care (Skilbeck et al. 2002). They spend time with patients and their families, helping them come to terms with an array of complex emotional and practical problems, facilitating communication, giving information and advice about treatments and also offering expertise in controlling pain and other distressing symptoms. These nurses are equipped with specialist skills to assess the complex palliative care needs of patients referred to the service. However, Bliss et al. (2000) found that referral to services is dependent upon the individual who initiates it and, although unintentional, may result in a form of gate-keeping with patients and carers not receiving services relevant to their needs.

The author is presently employed as a community palliative care clinical nurse specialist and in a recent study, as part of an MSc degree, set out to identify the triggers that motivate district nurses to refer patients to the service. The topic selected for the study resulted from observation within the author's clinical practice, where it was noted that district nurse referral patterns to the specialist nursing service were very inconsistent. Some district nurses refer regularly to the service, whilst others rarely refer. This raised the possibility that factors other than 'patient need' influenced referrals. The study incorporated semi-structured interviews with district nurses and the results of the research revealed a very apparent lack of knowledge regarding the role of the community palliative care clinical nurse specialist. A subsequent literature review also indicated that other authors had identified similar observations (Clark et al. 2002; Ahmed et al. 2004). As a consequence, the author has been afforded a valuable opportunity to produce a written text for community nurses, other members of the primary health care team and professionals involved in palliative care, on the role of the community palliative care clinical nurse specialist.

Palliative care is the active, total care of patients and their families by a multidisciplinary team; at a time when the patient's disease is no longer responsive to curative treatment and life expectancy is relatively short (Twycross 2003). The aim of palliative care is to provide support and care for patients and their families so that they can live as fully and comfortably as possible. Whilst many nursing texts discuss the challenges of palliative care in the home, few examine the role of the community palliative care clinical nurse specialist. This book hopes to provide its readers with a clear understanding of that role and the potential benefits that their knowledge and specialist skills can bring to the primary health care team.

The book is divided into three sections: professionals, patients and carers. The first section discusses the roles and contributions made by other members of the primary health care team, in particular, the pivotal role of the district nurse in caring for patients with palliative care needs. The text then examines the role of the community palliative care clinical nurse specialist. This role not only incorporates care to patients and their families, but also provides a source of professional support to other members of the primary health care team.

The psychosocial support needed by patients receiving palliative care is the subject of the second section. The text explores the community palliative care clinical nurse specialist's role in relation to complex psychological as well as practical problems surrounding a life-limiting illness. For example, the diverse issues involved in dealing with treatments, information needs, emotional demands and facing death will be explored. The use of case studies allows the reader a further insight into the complex needs of patients and their families. The role of the community palliative care clinical nurse specialist includes assessment of pain and symptom control. This is an important aspect of the role and involves liaising and negotiating with the primary care team to ensure optimum patient comfort. However, the text does not discuss symptom management, as there are many nursing and medical books on that subject, but instead concentrates on the complex support and information needs of seriously ill patients and their families. The text encompasses not only the patient's journey, but also that of the family during the illness trajectory and into the bereavement period.

The final section looks at the needs of the family and carers and the support that the community palliative care clinical nurse specialist can offer to these individuals. Included in this segment are the complex issues faced by carers in relation to the changing roles within the family, their children and impending death and bereavement. The assessment of the family is viewed as important to the management of the patient with palliative care needs (Payne et al. 2004); however, the core members of the primary health care team may struggle to fulfil family and carer needs due to time constraints and other demands from within primary care. It is therefore essential to utilise the expertise of other members of the primary health care team. The community palliative care clinical nurse specialist is in a unique position to be able to offer support to the patient with complex needs, and his or her family, not only during the patient's illness, but also into the bereavement period.

According to Bestall et al. (2004) the decision to refer a patient to specialist palliative care services relies upon the knowledge and expertise of the professional that the patient consults. It is therefore imperative that community nurses and others within the primary health care team are aware of the role of the community palliative care clinical nurse specialist. This book will help to inform and educate, to provide a stimulating resource for all professionals and students interested in palliative care and subsequently to improve the care of patients and their families in the community setting.

References

Ahmed N, Bestall JC, Ahmedzai SH, Payne S, Clark D, Noble B (2004) Systematic review of the problems and issues of accessing specialist palliative care by patients, carers and health and social care professionals. *Palliative Medicine* 18 (6), 525–542.

Bestall JC, Ahmed N, Ahmedzai SH, Payne SA, Noble B, Clark D (2004) Access and referral to specialist palliative care: patients' and professionals' experiences. *International Journal of Palliative Nursing* 10 (8), 381–389.

Bliss J, Cowley S, While A (2000) Interprofessional working in palliative care in the community: a review of the literature. *Journal of Interprofessional Care* 14 (3), 281–290.

Clark D, Seymour J, Douglas HR, et al. (2002) Clinical nurse specialists in palliative care. Part 2: Explaining diversity in the organisation and costs of Macmillan nursing services. *Palliative Medicine* 16 (5), 375–385.

Payne S, Seymour J, Ingleton C (eds) (2004) *Palliative Care Nursing: Principles and Evidence for Practice.* Open University, Maidenhead.

Skilbeck J, Corner J, Bath P, et al. (2002) Clinical nurse specialists in palliative care. Part 1: A description of the Macmillan nurse caseload. *Palliative Medicine* 16 (4), 285–296.

Twycross R (2003) *Introducing Palliative Care*, 4th edn. Radcliffe Medical Press, Abingdon.

Section I
Professionals

Community Palliative Care: The Team

Introduction

The patient receiving palliative care at home may potentially be in contact with a wide variety of professionals and support services. This chapter explores the concept of palliative care and briefly examines the roles of health care professionals within the community setting. Particular attention is given to the pivotal work of the district nurse in caring for patients with palliative care needs at home. Specialist palliative care and its various functions within the community are introduced, highlighting the collaborative working between primary health care teams and the specialist services.

Palliative care

Palliative care is an important part of the every-day work of most health care professionals, whether they work in the hospital or community setting. The word 'palliative' originates from the Latin *pallium*, a cloak. In palliative care, symptoms are 'cloaked' with treatments whose primary aim is to promote comfort. The more modern definition in the Oxford mini-dictionary may prove easier to understand: *reducing bad effects*. But what is palliative care? The recognised World Health Organisation (1990) definition describes palliative care as '*the active total care of patients whose disease is not responsive to curative treatment*'. Palliative care is considered, in most definitions, to incorporate the physical, psychological, social and spiritual aspects of care and is orientated to patients who have a non-curative condition. Palliative care should not be confused with terminal care, as many patients have palliative care needs from the time of their diagnosis and require ongoing palliative care for many months or years (Costello 2004). The aim of palliative care is to assist patients and their families through the physical and emotional traumas of life-threatening illness and to support them in that journey. Palliative care is not limited to cancer or even to the terminal stages of illness; it can last for years, and can be applied to any life-threatening disease, though it is most often associated with cancer. Palliative care is not an alternative to other care, but is a complementary and essential component of total patient care.

Developments in palliative care have been dramatic. Today, much of our understanding and knowledge of the subject has grown through the work of the hospice movement (Faull 1998). During the 1960s the first tentative steps were taken in the United Kingdom towards the growth of modern palliative care. The first hospice, incorporating research and teaching, was founded in 1967 by Cecily Saunders in London. The subsequent expansion of the hospice movement illustrated the value of 'care not cure'-focused institutions, with priority given to symptom control (Turton and Orr 1993). In due course, the1980s saw the speciality of palliative medicine being formally recognised. This allowed for not only an improvement in care for patients with palliative needs, but also research into best practice and ongoing multidisciplinary education. Although modern hospices and 'palliative care' embody a relatively young concept, their effects have been enormous and as a result many patients have been enabled to maintain a good quality of life, to die peacefully, and to know that their families are supported after their deaths (Addington-Hall and Higginson 2001).

Since the beginning of the modern hospice movement, emphasis has been on care of the patient with cancer, but clinicians are realising that the principles of palliative care extend beyond malignant disease to the care of patients with diseases such as congestive cardiac failure, chronic obstructive pulmonary disease, stroke, motor neurone disease, etc. The illness trajectory for some non-malignant diseases may be many years and the patient and his/her family will require ongoing symptom control and support, comparable to the cancer patient. Therefore the provision of palliative care is now based on need and not diagnosis, ensuring that appropriate care is available to all and not just to cancer patients.

At the beginning of the 20th century, the majority of people died at home with the care being given by the family, but medicine has changed considerably over the last 100 years. Developments in medical science and new treatments moved the focus of care away from the patients' homes into the hospitals; correspondingly, the number of people dying at home has fallen progressively. Figures reveal that the home death rate is now low (23% for patients with cancer, 19% for all deaths) and the hospital death rate is high (55% for patients with cancer, 66% of all deaths) (Thomas 2003). However, patients with cancer, for example, spend over 90% of their last year of life at home (Addington-Hall and McCarthy 1995) and irrespective of where a patient dies, the emphasis has to be on caring for that patient and family at home during the patient's illness. The main location of palliative care therefore remains in the community, under the direction of the primary health care team.

Community palliative care services

Caring for seriously ill patients within their own homes can prove difficult and challenging to the health professionals involved; especially when the illness is progressing and there are the added complexities of distressing symptoms, emotional issues to address and family members to support. However, given the choice and a supportive family, most patients would want to be nursed at home during their illness and to die at home (Palmer and Howarth 2005). The aim of palliative care in the home is to have a well-supported family and ensure the patient is comfortable and able to deal with his or her approaching death. The patient may require assistance to manage not only physical, psychological, social and spiritual needs, but also legal and financial issues that may have to be addressed (Abu-Saad and Courtens 2001). This requires the skills of many professionals working together as a team to achieve the desired outcome.

Multidisciplinary team working lies at the heart of palliative care and involves many individuals working together with a common goal. Functioning as a team, the professionals can provide continuous and integrated supportive care. Today's patients and their families have increasingly high expectations of the health care services and what professionals should offer. Therefore, when the needs of the patient and family require ongoing visits from a number of disciplines, optimal care is given when the health care providers collaborate as a coordinated team. As such, the palliative care team requires excellent communication skills, an understanding of each other's abilities and an acceptance of 'blurred' role boundaries. This approach will support most patients and their families with a sense of security, consistency and comfort (Ingham and Coyle 1997).

Providing support for the family is an important role for the team, as carer fatigue is often the main factor in the hospitalisation of patients towards the end of their life. In order to sustain a patient at home, it is essential to consider the family carer as a member of the team, and consideration should be given to the carer's views and opinions, as well as to the patient. There is no 'typical' team in community palliative care; the composition is dependent on 'patient need' and the skills available to meet those needs. The patient receiving palliative care at home may potentially be in contact with a wide variety of professionals. For example, as well as the general practitioner and district nurse (who will be discussed later), the patient may need the services of the physiotherapist, occupational therapist, social services, dietician and Marie Curie nurses.

Physiotherapist

The role of the physiotherapist in palliative care is different from the therapist in a rehabilitation team; rather than attempting to improve function, the aim will be to maximise the patient's weakening resources, through problem solving and emotional support (Doyle et al. 1998). The community physiotherapist plays a significant role in the non-pharmacological relief of symptoms, improving patient mobility and as a specialist resource in the management of lymphoedema. The therapist may have contact with the patient in the home, at a symptom control clinic or in the day care setting. Physiotherapists have a particularly important part to play in managing the patient with breathlessness (Doyle and Jeffrey 2000); they can teach relaxation, breathing techniques and give assistance to those having difficulty expectorating. They also give advice to patients and their carers on lifting and transferring, or recommend appropriate walking aids to maximise mobility. As mentioned earlier, in many instances, they have specialist knowledge of the management of lymphoedema, which can be a debilitating and distressing condition. They can advise on massage or appropriate stockings or sleeves for limbs affected by lymphoedema and act as a resource for community nursing colleagues. In palliative care, physiotherapy includes the setting of achievable goals and aims to improve quality of life and encourage independence.

Occupational therapist

The role and contribution of community occupational therapists in palliative care is both varied and challenging. They play a vital role in providing adaptive equipment for the home. They approach the patient's problems as they arise and assist in the provision of equipment as appropriate (Cooper 1998). This can enable patients receiving palliative care to not only maintain a safer environment, but also retain independence for as long as possible. The ability to carry out normal daily living activities is often the main objective for patients with a life-threatening illness (Kealey and McIntyre 2005); occupational therapists can assess patients to determine their abilities for independent living and provide equipment and adaptations as necessary. They can advise on the provision of aids such as rails, ramps, commodes and raised toilet seats. Giving practical advice and support to families and carers is also an important aspect of their role and can be invaluable in helping families to adjust to the ever-changing needs of the patient.

Social services

The aim of social work in palliative care is to help patients and their families with the social and personal problems of illness, disability and impending death (Doyle et al. 1998). Social workers are usually responsible for co-ordinating the package of social care at home to meet the needs of the patient and family. Social services provide for individuals with palliative care needs through social workers, home carers, meals on wheels, emergency alarm systems, etc. The primary health care team work very closely with the social work department and increasingly rely on them for providing assistance with personal care, meal provision, medication prompting, financial assessment and carer support. The social worker can also advise on child care issues and housing difficulties. The aim of social services is to allow patients to remain as independent as possible, within a supportive environment with their own families.

Dietician

The dietician's knowledge and skills can make a valuable contribution to the team caring for patients with palliative care needs. The inability to eat and enjoy food is just one of the losses for a patient dealing with a life-threatening illness. Effective management of nutrition-related problems can improve quality of life; significant weight loss may lead to weakness and lethargy (Hill and Hart 2001). The dietician can assess patients and give advice to patients and their families on diet and nutritional supplements. The carers may also benefit from explanation and guidance to allay fears and concerns regarding the dietary intake of the seriously ill patient.

Marie Curie nurses

The Marie Curie nursing service was established in the United Kingdom in 1958 to care for patients in their own homes (Higginson and Wilkinson 2002). The service provides direct nursing care and support to patients and carers by providing overnight care and also day 'sits' to allow exhausted family members respite. Marie Curie nurses are experienced registered nurses and healthcare assistants who receive induction training before working with patients. The nurses are not specialists in palliative care, but deliver essential nursing care to the patients usually in accordance with the district nursing care plan. They can monitor symptoms, give medication, provide support and allow carers much needed respite. Referral to the service is through the primary health care team, usually the district nurse. They are organised and funded by the nationwide charity Marie Curie Cancer Care, in partnership with the NHS.

As the above demonstrates, in order to meet the diverse needs of patients, it is necessary to utilise a range of disciplines. The roles discussed are by no means the complete list of professionals that a patient may encounter in the community, but merely those more commonly involved in palliative care. In reality, however, only a few individuals will be providing the majority of the care. The key professionals within the primary health care team caring for the patient at home are the general practitioner and the district nurse. According to Hull et al. (1989), when a patient is very ill, the first need is for expert nursing care and the second need is for an understanding doctor, skilled in communication and symptom control. Palliative care is at its very best when the skills of the different professionals are combined.

General practitioner

Ultimate responsibility for the overall medical care of patients in the community rests with the general practitioner (Jatsch 2002). The majority of general practitioners now work in multi-partner practices, allowing for greater flexibility, but potentially less continuity for patients (Barnett 2002). With the changes in the organisation of primary care and the use of out-of-hours cooperatives, there is less emphasis on home visiting and continuity becomes even more difficult to provide (Doyle and Jeffrey 2000). The general practitioner is, however, in a unique position, as he/she may have considerable previous knowledge about the patient and his or her family and therefore may understand the dynamics within the patient's home to a greater extent than any other professional within primary care. Indeed, many families regard the general practitioner as the professional who has cared for them over many years and with whom they have built a relationship of trust. In today's health service, however, this relationship may be more difficult for general practitioners to establish and maintain due to the ever-increasing workload demands within primary care.

Taking into account this increasing workload and the time and resources required caring for a patient at home with palliative care needs, do general practitioners today envisage their role as incorporating palliative care? In a study of London general practitioners by Burt et al. (2006), the majority of general practitioners (72%) who participated agreed that palliative care was a central part of their role. Within the primary health care team, the general practitioner is usually seen to have a key role (in conjunction with the district nurse) in coordinating palliative care and appropriately referring onto other services when needs arise. According to Costello (2004) the quality of care provided by the general practitioner and other members of the primary health care team determines the ability of the family to cope at home during this traumatic time. Though individual general practitioners rarely have more than a handful of patients requiring palliative care at one time, their role in supportive care and accessing other services cannot be overstated (Brennan 2004). They must be prepared to take time to foresee and alleviate potential problems and be adept in communicating with patients and their families. General practitioners require a good knowledge of symptom control, but it is also essential for them to understand their limitations in terms of both palliative skills and time constraints (Jatsch 2002). Their role is to enable the patient with palliative care needs to carry on living, at times for many months or years, and, where appropriate, provide medication to ensure relief of symptoms, thereby maintaining quality of life until the patient dies (Charlton 2002).

District nurse

District nurses are the largest group of community nurses in the United Kingdom (Bryans and McIntosh 2000; Kennedy 2002) and responsibility for assessing and planning how patients' and families' needs are met in the home constitutes a basic component of their role (Kennedy 2002). They can trace their roots back to the mid 19th century, when William Rathbone provided the first fully trained hospital nurse, Mrs Robinson, to care for the sick poor in their own homes in Liverpool. At that time, district nurses had to contend with welfare issues such as poor sanitation, unemployment and overcrowding: their concerns were not only for the patient, but also for the health of the family. Through the decades, district nursing services have been continually developing in response to the changing needs of the community (Boran and Clarridge 2005), and the traditional work of district nurses has been redefined and their remit has now expanded to include, for example, nurse prescribing and the assessment and management of patients with long-term conditions. Today's district nurse provides a modern service which is accessible, meets the needs of patients and carers and is delivered within the patient's own home.

District nurses are registered nurses who have undertaken additional post registration education, now at both degree and post graduate level, in order to gain a recognised district nurse qualification. They are highly skilled nurses and lead teams of community staff nurses and nursing assistants, coordinating nursing care for those patients within a geographical area or within a practice population. Practical nursing at home is not the same as in a hospital setting. The situations district nurses often encounter within the community can be complex and nursing activity is therefore likely to be influenced by a number of factors including social circumstances, the environment, resources available and the expectations of the patient and family. The district nurse provides nursing care to patients through direct access from self referral and also receives referrals from other members of the primary health care team and secondary care. Early referral to the district nursing service of patients with a life-threatening illness permits the nurse to assess the needs of the patient and carer and allow time to 'get to know' the family. This early contact is important for establishing relationships with patients and their carers before the time when intimate care is needed and death approaches (Griffiths et al. 2007).

The district nursing work-load has changed considerably in recent years as a result of changes in community care legislation and they are now providing less personal hygiene care, with more emphasis on assessment and skilled nursing, such as palliative care (Barclay 2001). The district nurse is indeed the palliative care linchpin of the primary care team (Barnett 2002) and can be considered the 'key' person in the provision of palliative care in the home (McIlfatrick and

Curran 2000). The district nurse spends a considerable amount of time caring for patients, not only with cancer, but also with other chronic illnesses, and her knowledge and expertise can ensure that all individuals with a life-threatening illness, irrespective of diagnosis, receive effective palliative care. Dunne et al. (2005) report that although research examining the role of district nurses in palliative care is sparse, they are identified as providing practical nursing care, symptom management and emotional support for patients and their families. Their nursing support is particularly important to families, both for reassurance and to alleviate the physical burden of caring.

District nurses view themselves as having a central and valued role in palliative care, where the focus of their work will be the nursing assessment of the patient, meeting basic nursing needs, control of symptoms and support to the family. However, Simpson (2003) states that district nurses often lack the confidence to support patients and their families at home due to insufficient training, whilst a study by Wright (2002) has highlighted concerns that they may not have the necessary skills to provide such care effectively. She examined the district nurses' perspective in caring for patients receiving palliative care and found nurses lacking the skills to communicate with patients about emotional issues such as death and dying. Dunne et al. (2005) also found district nurses feeling inadequate and helpless in dealing particularly with children and young people in the family and as a result tending to exclude them from conversations. This may lead to the district nurse using 'blocking' strategies to avoid certain difficult topics. The difficulties that district nurses have in communicating with some patients receiving palliative care suggest that there is a gap in their knowledge and skills. This deficit in their patient care indicates that referral onto other services would be appropriate, in particular, the community palliative care clinical nurse specialist. It is important for district nurses to be aware of their own limitations and refer patients to the most appropriate service as needs arise, or the situation in the home changes. This requires a clear understanding of the services available within their own community, regarding not only skills and knowledge, but also access to these services (Bliss et al. 2000).

As mentioned previously, a small-scale research study undertaken by the author (Aitken 2006) cast some doubt on the district nurses' role in referring onto other services when difficulties arose. The study set out to identify the triggers that motivate district nurses to refer patients to the community palliative care clinical nurse specialist: the topic selected resulted from observation within the researcher's clinical practice, when it was noted that referral patterns to the community palliative care clinical nurse specialist were very inconsistent. Other authors, namely Beaver et al. (2000) and Hughes (2004), had noted that cancer patients in particular had contact primarily with the district nurses and that they may potentially act as gate-keepers to other services. In order to provide effective palliative care in the home, the district nurses require an awareness of services available to patients and their families, but it became apparent in the author's research that there was a lack of knowledge amongst the district nurses regarding the role of the community palliative care clinical nurse specialist. This lack of knowledge relating to these specialist nurses has been affirmed previously by several authors (Graves and Nash 1993; Clark et al. 2002; Ahmed et al. 2004). Skilbeck and Seymour (2002) report that some staff respond to palliative care in a reactive manner, calling the community palliative care clinical nurse specialist to sort out a crisis. Indeed it was acknowledged by several of the district nurses in the author's study that they contact the specialist nurse when 'they were out of their depth' or 'when struggling with the patient'. This late intervention cannot be compatible with good palliative care. Palliative home care is a team effort (Wong et al. 2004) and district nurses need to utilise other services to meet the complex needs of their patients and their families.

Despite the findings of some authors questioning the knowledge and skills of the district nurses, or the perceived reluctance to refer onto other services, the district nursing team members carry out a valued and central role in the management of patients with palliative care needs. They visit patients in their own homes, carry out nursing assessments, produce care plans in conjunction with the patient and family and provide much of the day-to-day nursing care required. This individualised patient-centred approach is vital in order to plan and deliver care that is structured to the needs of the patient and family (Henry 2001). This allows patients the choice of where they want to be nursed and eventually die, knowing that their family will also be supported by the skilled district nursing team.

Specialist palliative care services

Palliative care now encompasses a wide range of specialist services and has made great strides forward since Dame Cicely Saunders opened St Christopher's hospice in London. Over the past four decades the hospice movement has been at the forefront of specialist palliative care provision in the United Kingdom, with the number of hospices and specialist palliative care teams having increased considerably in the intervening years. This growth has also led to improvements in the care that can be offered to patients and their families. These teams have gained their skills and knowledge mainly from working with patients dying from cancer, but this knowledge can be readily transferable to patients with non-cancer diagnoses (Palmer and Howarth 2005). Increasingly intervention from the specialist team is at an earlier stage in the patient's illness trajectory, where there may be difficult symptoms or complex psychological or social issues to manage (Barnett 2002).

Specialist palliative care has a variety of functions: as a resource of specialist expertise to the primary health care team or hospital staff, to offer education to other health professionals, to undertake research and to provide direct care to patients and families with complex needs. Specialist palliative care is provided by a multidisciplinary team of health professionals who have specialist qualifications and experience in the care of patients and their families who are living with a life-threatening illness and face impending death. Their involvement is most appropriate for patients with complex and difficult to manage symptoms or needs. According to Barnett (2002), specialist palliative care services are involved with 50% or more of all cancer patients who are terminally ill, but their remit is increasingly extending to those with non-malignant diagnoses. These professionals may work in specialist community palliative care teams, specialist day care centres, within the hospital palliative care team or hospice setting.

Hospital palliative care teams

Although many patients with a life-threatening illness spend the majority of their final year at home (Addington-Hall and McCarthy 1995), they may require hospital admission from time to time. This may be for treatments, symptom control and assessment of symptoms or end of life care. Their admission and ongoing care within the hospital may necessitate referral to the hospital palliative care team. The core members of the hospital palliative care team are clinical nurse specialists and consultants in palliative medicine. Most palliative care teams in the hospital setting are working in an advisory capacity and do not take over patient care; however, the benefits of such an advisory team cannot be overstated. Their aim is to empower their generalist colleagues to provide a high standard of care to the patients. They have a flexible response to referrals and may have direct contact with the patient or simply give telephone advice to colleagues. The assessment of a patient by the palliative care team at times reveals significant problems that the referring team may not have identified (Butler 2004). The team can have several roles, including assessment of patient need, giving specialist advice on pain and symptom control, monitoring palliative care management, education, support for patients, families and carers, as well as liaison with community colleagues.

Hospice inpatient units

The size of inpatient hospices across the United Kingdom varies greatly, the average unit accommodating 15 beds (Doyle 1998), with many having been built and funded as a result of public appeal (Barnett 2002). The larger units, although still called hospices, will probably be specialist palliative care units, comprising one or more consultants in palliative medicine, with other junior medical staff in attendance (Doyle and Jeffrey 2000). Admission to these inpatient units is considered for symptom control, end of life care or assessment and rehabilitation.

Their staffing consists of multidisciplinary teams of medical and nursing personnel, physiotherapists, occupational therapists, pharmacists, social workers, chaplains, volunteers, complementary therapists, etc. and most have a higher staff ratio of qualified nurses (Woof et al. 1998) than acute inpatient units. The staff will all have qualifications in palliative care or have had experience in caring for patients with palliative care needs. The accommodation generally will deliver an atmosphere of calm, in a welcoming environment, allowing for privacy and a sense of security (Woof et al. 1998). The hospice model of care was developed to meet the needs of the dying and their families and encompasses skilled and compassionate palliative care interventions regardless of prognosis or closeness to death (Coyle 2006).

Specialist community palliative care teams

The first community specialist palliative care team was established from St Christopher's hospice in London in 1969, with support from the Department of Health (Hansford 2004). Today specialist palliative care teams in the community may be solely community based, or may be associated with hospice or hospital teams (Barnett 2002). The team usually consists of community palliative care clinical nurse specialists and a consultant in palliative medicine; access will be available to other disciplines, for example, social workers, physiotherapists, occupational therapists and dieticians. The specialists can provide support not only for patients and their families within the home, but also to the primary health care team. Their involvement within primary care also extends to information, advice and education, on a one-to-one basis or more formally. For many patients, a community palliative care clinical nurse specialist, working with the primary health care team, may be the only part of specialist palliative care they will need (Woof et al. 1998).

Specialist nurses

When providing palliative care nursing services it is important to explain the difference between a nurse working in a specialty and a specialist nurse. Nurses working in specialties such as palliative care give everyday basic care to patients whether it is in their home or a hospital setting (Elias 1999). They may have considerable knowledge and experience in that subject, but are not specialist nurses. Specialist nurses are registered nurses who have undertaken and completed higher and advanced level education programmes in their chosen area of practice, for example, palliative care. The role of the community palliative care clinical nurse specialist will be described in detail in the next chapter.

Specialist day care centre

This is a rapidly expanding area of specialist palliative care and the numbers of specialist day care centres has grown in the United Kingdom, from 11 in 1980 to 243 in 2002 (Kennett 2004). The day care centre offers physical and emotional support to patients living at home with palliative care needs. These centres typically cater for 10–15 patients per day (Twycross 2003) and aim to promote rehabilitation and help the patients in gaining some independence in daily living. The centre also provides social support and can give much needed respite to carers. Most of these centres will offer physiotherapy, occupational therapy, complementary therapies, medical review, monitoring of symptoms, symptom control clinics, lymphoedema clinics, advice and information, nursing care and many other services. Some centres also provide day care facilities for supportive procedures such as blood transfusions and bisphosphonate infusions.

Specialist palliative care in the community should be seen as complementing, not replacing, the services provided by other health care professionals within primary care. There is no intention to take over from the patient's own general practitioner or district nursing team, but to work collaboratively for the benefit of the patient and family. The aim is to care for those patients and their families with physical, psychological, social or spiritual needs that are difficult to manage. Specialist palliative care teams are well aware that patients and their families want to be looked after by their own general practitioner and district nurses, and therefore the role of the specialist team is to support them and enable this to take place (Doyle and Jeffrey 2000).

Key Points

- Palliative care incorporates the physical, psychological, social and spiritual aspects of care and is orientated to patients who have a non-curative condition.
- The aim of palliative care is to assist the patient and family through the physical and emotional traumas of life-threatening illness and support them in that journey.
- Caring for seriously ill patients within their own homes can prove difficult and challenging to the health professionals involved, especially when the illness is progressing and there are complex symptoms or emotional issues to be addressed.
- Multidisciplinary team working lies at the heart of palliative care and involves many individuals working together with a common goal.
- Communication between professionals is an essential element of effective palliative care.
- The district nurse is the palliative care linchpin of the primary care team and can be considered the key person in the provision of palliative care in the home.
- Specialist palliative care has a variety of functions: as a resource for health professionals, education, research and to provide direct care to patients with complex or difficult to manage symptoms.
- Specialist palliative care in the community should be seen as complementing, not replacing, the services provided by other health care professionals within the primary care team.

Useful resources

Charlton R (ed) (2002) *Primary Palliative Care: Death, Dying and Bereavement*. Radcliffe Medical Press, Abingdon.

Doyle D, Jeffrey D (2000) *Palliative Care in the Home*. Oxford University Press, Oxford.

Palmer E, Howarth J (2005) *Palliative Care for the Primary Care Team*. Quay Books, London.

Thomas K (2003) *Caring for the Dying at Home: Companions on the Journey*. Radcliffe Medical Press, Abingdon.

References

Abu-Saad H, Courtens A (2001) Models of palliative care. In: Abu-Saad H (ed) *Evidence-Based Palliative Care: Across the Life Span*, pp 14–24. Blackwell Science, Oxford.

Addington-Hall J, Higginson I (eds) (2001) *Palliative Care for Non-Cancer Patients*. Oxford University Press, Oxford.

Addington-Hall J, McCarthy M (1995) Regional study of care for the dying: method and sample characteristics. *Palliative Medicine* 9 (1), 27–35.

Ahmed N, Bestall JC, Ahmedzai SH, Payne S, Clark D, Noble B (2004) Systemic review of the problems and issues of accessing specialist palliative care by patients, carers and health and social care professionals. *Palliative Medicine* 18 (6), 525–542.

Aitken A (2006) District nurses' triggers for referral of patients to the Macmillan nurse. *British Journal of Community Nursing* 11 (3), 100–107.

Barclay S (2001) Palliative care for non-cancer patients: a UK perspective from primary care. In: Addington-Hall, J Higginson I (eds) *Palliative Care for Non-Cancer Patients*, pp 172–188. Oxford University Press, Oxford.

Barnett M (2002) The development of palliative care within primary care. In: Charlton R (ed) *Primary Palliative Care: Death, Dying and Bereavement*, pp 1–14. Radcliffe Medical Press, Abingdon.

Beaver K, Luker KA, Woods S (2000) Primary care services received during terminal illness. *International Journal of Palliative Nursing* 6 (5), 220–227.

Bliss J, Cowley S, While A (2000) Interprofessional working in palliative care in the community: a review of the literature. *Journal of Interprofessional Care* 14 (3), 281–290.

Boran S, Clarridge A (2005) Contemporary issues in district nursing. In: Sines D, Appleby F, Frost M (eds) *Community Health Care Nursing*, 3rd edn, pp 146–159. Blackwell Publishing, Oxford.

Brennan J (2004) *Cancer in Context: A Practical Guide to Supportive Care*. Oxford University Press, Oxford.

Bryans A, McIntosh J (2000) The use of simulation interview and post-simulation interview to examine the knowledge involved in community nursing assessment practice. *Journal of Advanced Nursing* 31 (5), 1244–1251.

Burt J, Shipman C, White P, Addington-Hall J (2006) Roles, service knowledge and priorities in provision of palliative care: a postal survey of London GPs. *Palliative Medicine* 20 (5), 487–492.

Butler C (2004) The hospital palliative care team. In: Sykes N, Edmonds P, Wiles J (eds) *Management of Advanced Disease*, 4th edn, pp 530–537. Arnold, London.

Charlton R (ed) (2002) *Primary Palliative Care: Death, Dying and Bereavement*. Radcliffe Medical Press, Abingdon.

Clark D, Seymour J, Douglas HR, et al. (2002) Clinical nurse specialists in palliative care. Part 2: Explaining diversity in the organisation and costs of Macmillan nursing services. *Palliative Medicine* 16 (5), 375–385.

Cooper J (ed) (1998) *Occupational Therapy in Oncology and Palliative Care*. Whurr, London.

Costello J (2004) *Nursing the Dying Patient: Caring in Different Contexts*. Palgrave Macmillan, Basingstoke.

Coyle N (2006) Introduction to palliative nursing care. In: Ferrel BR, Coyle N (eds) *Textbook of Palliative Nursing*, 2nd edn, pp 5–11. Oxford University Press, Oxford.

Doyle D (1998) The provision of palliative care. In: Doyle D, Hanks GWC, MacDonald N (eds) *Oxford Textbook of Palliative Medicine*, 2nd edn, pp 41–53. Oxford University Press, Oxford.

Doyle D, Jeffrey D (2000) *Palliative Care in the Home*. Oxford University Press, Oxford.

Doyle D, Hanks GWC, MacDonald N (eds) (1998) *Oxford Textbook of Palliative Medicine*, 2nd edn. Oxford University Press, Oxford.

Dunne K, Sullivan K, Kernohan G (2005) Palliative care for patients with cancer: district nurses' experiences. *Journal of Advanced Nursing* 50 (4), 372–380.

Elias E (1999) Palliative care. In: Littlewood J (ed) *Current Issues in Community Nursing: Specialist Practice in Primary Health Care*, pp 119–144. Churchill Livingstone, Edinburgh.

Faull C (1998) The history and principles of palliative care. In: Faull C, Carter Y, Woof R (eds) *Handbook of Palliative Care*, pp 1–12. Blackwell Science, Oxford.

Graves D, Nash A (1993) Referring patients for domiciliary care. *Nursing Standard* 7 (24), 25–28.

Griffiths J, Ewing G, Rogers M, et al. (2007) Supporting cancer patients with palliative care needs: district nurses' role perceptions. *Cancer Nursing* 30 (2), 156–162.

Hansford P (2004) The home care team. In: Sykes N, Edmonds P, Wiles J (eds) *Management of Advanced Disease*, 4th edn, pp 522–529. Arnold, London.

Henry C (2001) Death, dying and bereavement. In: Watson NA, Wilkinson C (eds) *Nursing in Primary Care: A Handbook for Students*, pp 307–336. Palgrave, Basingstoke.

Higginson IJ, Wilkinson S (2002) Marie Curie nurses: enabling patients with cancer to die at home. *British Journal of Community Nursing* 7 (5), 240–244.

Hill D, Hart K (2001) A practical approach to nutritional support for patients with advanced cancer. *International Journal of Palliative Nursing* 7 (7), 317–321.

Hughes L (2004) Palliative care in the community. *Primary Health Care* 14 (6), 27–31.

Hull R, Ellis M, Sargent V (1989) *Teamwork in Palliative Care*. Radcliffe Medical Press, Abingdon.

Ingham JM, Coyle N (1997) Teamwork in end-of-life care: a nurse-physician perspective on introducing physicians to palliative care concepts. In: Clark D, Hockley J, Ahmedzai S (eds) *Facing Death: New Themes in Palliative Care*, pp 255–274. Open University Press, Buckingham.

Jatsch W (2002) Role of the primary health care team in palliative care. In: Charlton R (ed) *Primary Palliative Care: Death, Dying and Bereavement*, pp 131–142. Radcliffe Medical Press, Abingdon.

Kealey P, McIntyre I (2005) An evaluation of the domiciliary occupational therapy service in palliative cancer care in a community trust: a patient and carer's perspective. *European Journal of Cancer Care* 14 (3), 232–243.

Kennedy C (2002) The work of district nurses: first assessment visits. *Journal of Advanced Nursing* 40 (6), 710–720.

Kennett C (2004) Specialist palliative day care. In: Sykes N, Edmonds P, Wiles J (eds) *Management of Advanced Disease*, 4th edn, pp 538–544. Arnold, London.

McIlfatrick S, Curran CI (2000) District nurses' perceptions of palliative care services: part 2. *International Journal of Palliative Nursing* 6 (1), 32–38.

Palmer E, Howarth J (2005) *Palliative Care for the Primary Care Team*. Quay Books, London.

Simpson M (2003) Developing education and support for community nurses: principles and practice of palliative care. *Nursing Management* 9 (9), 9–12.

Skilbeck J, Seymour J (2002) Meeting complex needs: an analysis of Macmillan nurses' work with patients. *International Journal of Palliative Nursing* 8 (12), 574–582.

Thomas K (2003) *Caring for the Dying at Home: Companions on the Journey.* Radcliffe Medical Press, Abingdon.

Turton P, Orr J (1993) *Learning to Care in the Community*, 2nd edn. Edward Arnold, London.

Twycross R (2003) *Introducing Palliative Care*, 4th edn. Radcliffe Medical Press, Abingdon.

Wong FKY, Liu CF, Szeto Y, Sham M, Chan T (2004) Health problems encountered by dying patients receiving palliative home care until death. *Cancer Nursing* 27 (3), 244–251.

Woof R, Carter Y, Harrison B, Faull C, Nyatanga B (1998) Terminal care and dying. In: Faull C, Carter Y, Woof R (eds) *Handbook of Palliative Care*, pp 307–332. Blackwell Science, Oxford.

World Health Organisation (1990) *Cancer Pain Relief and Palliative Care.* World Health Organisation, Geneva.

Wright K (2002) Caring for the terminally ill: the district nurse's perspective. *British Journal of Nursing* 11 (18), 1180–1185.

The Role of the Community Palliative Care Clinical Nurse Specialist

Introduction

This chapter is written to provide a clearer understanding of the role of the community palliative care clinical nurse specialist. These nurses are equipped with specialist skills to assess the complex palliative care needs of patients with a life-threatening condition. The text explores the five main functions of the clinical nurse specialist role and the added skills and knowledge that the specialist nurse can bring to the health care team. These nurses are available to support patients with cancer and other life-threatening illnesses from the time they are diagnosed and play an important role in the psychological support of patients and their families facing advanced disease.

Clinical nurse specialists

Clinical nurse specialists can be defined as experts in a particular field of nursing; possessing advanced education, linking theory to practice and ensuring that nursing care is research based and of a high standard. The concept of a specialist role in clinical nursing was first described by Reiter in 1943 (Bousfield 1997) who used the term 'nurse clinician' and described the role as a nurse who would be able to demonstrate and provide care, plan and supervise the care given by other nurses and act as staff consultant and educator. She later stated that the clinical nurse specialist should function as an expert practitioner and role model providing the highest quality of nursing care (Reiter 1966). The emergence of the clinical nurse specialist role can be related to advances in medical technology and the ensuing need for specialised and complex nursing care.

The clinical nurse specialist role was first pioneered in America in the 1960s, and was intended to keep expert nurses at the bedside; the role was slower to evolve in the United Kingdom, emerging a decade or so later, in the late1970s and early 1980s (Castledine 2003). Education to Master's or Doctorate level is required in America to practise as a clinical nurse specialist; but the role in the United Kingdom has not been clearly defined and is much debated (Llahana 2005). This debate has been ongoing for many years and there is considerable confusion between the clinical nurse specialist and other nursing specialities, for example, the nurse practitioner. This lack of clarity has manifested in discrepancies within the nursing profession with regard to specialist/advanced nursing titles, differing roles and the educational needs of these nurses.

In the United Kingdom, the idea of advanced practice, such as the clinical nurse specialist, was first discussed by the Royal College of Nursing in the 1970s following the Briggs Report (Department of Health and Social Security 1972). However, the role seems to have evolved on an individual basis, unplanned and reactive, determined by local service needs and not in accordance to any professional framework. In 1994, the United Kingdom Central Council (UKCC) produced the document 'Standards for Education and Practice Following Registration' and stated that specialist practice was at a higher level of practice than that required for initial registration and that those nurses with a first degree in their area of practice were specialist practitioners (Reveley et al. 2001). While this may be true, in the United Kingdom, unlike America, educational standards are less clearly specified for the clinical nurse specialist role and appear to depend more on clinical experience and management discretion (Llahana 2005).

This lack of clarity regarding the role, the responsibilities and the preparation for the role of clinical nurse specialist (Castledine and McGee 1998) has consequently resulted in a wide variance in the qualifications, education and clinical experience found within the clinical nurse specialists in the United Kingdom. It could be argued, however, that many nurses now working as clinical nurse specialists in the United Kingdom are indeed educated to Master's degree level similar to their American counterparts. In many instances, the nurses have undertaken this education as part of their ongoing professional development, rather than a requirement of their job description.

The implementation within the NHS of the Agenda for Change in 2005 aimed to evaluate nursing roles based on a nationally agreed Knowledge and Skills Framework (Department of Health 2004) and this indeed recommends a Master's degree for advanced practice, such as clinical nurse specialists. However, at the time of writing, the author is aware that the implementation of this framework is still in its infancy and the impact on nursing roles is still unknown.

The clinical nurse specialist's role

The clinical nurse specialist works mainly within the hospital setting in the United States of America. However, in the United Kingdom, clinical nurse specialists are working within both the secondary and primary care settings. But what constitutes their role? The United Kingdom Central Council for Nursing, Midwifery and Health Visiting (1998) identified seven components of what it termed 'higher practice': providing effective health care, improving quality and health outcome, evaluation and research, leading and developing practice, innovation and changing practice, developing self and others, and working across professional boundaries and organisational boundaries.

Unfortunately, the terminology of 'higher practice' can be misinterpreted and does not clearly identify the function of the clinical nurse specialist. Several other authors have defined the role of the clinical nurse specialist as incorporating five distinct areas of practice: clinical, research, consultative, education and leadership (Hamric and Spross 1989; Miller 1995; Bousfield 1997; Skilbeck et al. 2002; Llahana 2005). Each clinical nurse specialist will interpret his or her role uniquely depending on the needs of patients, staff, employing organisation, etc., but the basic components will be similar and will be discussed below.

Clinical expert

The provision of direct patient care has been a crucial element of the clinical nurse specialist role since its introduction in the 1960s. The role was introduced to provide expert care to patients with complex nursing needs, by skilled nurses at the bedside. The role has evolved through the decades and may now constitute direct or indirect care by the specialist on a day-to-day basis, episodically as needs arise, or through education of others to provide the care. The clinical nurse specialist, as an expert practitioner, will assess, plan, deliver and evaluate care at an advanced level and may identify more potential problems, as a result of her education and experience, than a less qualified nursing colleague (Koetters 1989). The function of the clinical nurse specialist as a role model cannot be overstated. The knowledge base of the clinical nurse specialist allows her to develop clinical protocols and standards for the management of patients with complex needs, to allow other nursing staff to execute the ongoing nursing care (Llahana 2005). The clinical nurse specialist will have up-to-date research knowledge and is therefore ideally placed to undertake audit on clinical practice. This should not only improve the nursing care of those patients with whom the specialist has direct intervention, but also improve the overall quality of nursing care.

Researcher

Involvement in research is a basic component of the clinical nurse specialist role, involving not only application of research findings into nursing practice, but also participation in the research process. If the aim of clinical nurse specialists is to enhance patient care, then research must be part of the role (Armstrong 1999). It will involve their awareness of current literature and research, assessing its reliability and validity, disseminating the research to colleagues and evaluating that research in nursing practice. The clinical nurse specialist requires critical thinking skills and problem solving abilities to carry out the research role. However, clinical nurse specialists' involvement in research will be determined by a number of factors, such as their interest and commitment to research, educational preparation, job description and the clinical setting (McGuire and Harwood 1989). The clinical nurse specialist is in a unique position to be able to bridge the gap between theory and practice and ensure that nursing care is of a high standard.

Consultant

Consultation is an important aspect of the clinical nurse specialist role, whether it takes place formally at the bedside or informally in the coffee-room. The aim of the consultation is to enhance the consultee's skill and knowledge in dealing with a current work difficulty and enable him/her to resolve comparable situations in the future (Armstrong 1999). These problems usually relate to the care and treatment of patients, and the clinical nurse specialist requires excellent communication skills, self awareness, interpersonal skills, as well as clinical expertise to address issues and function in this role. The enhanced knowledge and skills of the clinical nurse specialist permits her to provide advice on a wide range of topics relating to care of the patient with complex needs. The clinical nurse specialist in her role as consultant has to feel comfortable with a significant degree of autonomy, as many of the every-day decisions, problem solving and evaluation will be managed on her own (Barron 1989).

This can be a challenging and complex professional undertaking. The consultant element of the clinical nurse specialist role is influenced by many factors, including the needs of the patients and staff, the expertise of the staff, the goals and priorities of the health care unit and also the aims and objectives of the clinical nurse specialist (Barron 1989). However, the aim of the consultation will be to enhance knowledge, inspire confidence in the consultee to overcome the difficulties and ultimately enhance patient care.

Educator

Educational responsibilities are a traditional part of the clinical nurse specialists' role (Llahana 2005). They pass on information not only at the bedside, but also more formally at study days, post basic courses, lectures and talks. The audience may be fellow nurses, but increasingly education is multi-professional and will include medical colleagues, allied health professionals and personnel from social services. The teaching of health care students, at both pre and post graduate level, is an important aspect of the role, encouraging them to apply their knowledge to the complexities of health and illness (Priest 1989). The teaching role also incorporates instruction to patients and their families both at home and in the hospital setting, selecting the most appropriate method for each patient or situation. As a clinical expert and manager of complex patient situations, the clinical nurse specialist is in an ideal position to assume the role of educator, assisting patients and their families to understand their illness and help them navigate their way through the illness trajectory (Priest 1989).

Leader

The clinical nurse specialist has responsibility for innovation and change within her sphere of practice and has considerable influence in determining patient care. Developing new concepts of care, and re-examining and evaluating ongoing practice are all aspects of the leadership role (Armstrong 1999). The specialist's leadership skills will be demonstrated by caring for patients with complex needs and resolving their clinical problems (Gournic 1989), either through direct care or by supervising and influencing others. Leadership demands excellent organisational skills and the authority to guide professionals when required (Castledine and McGee 1998). This needs the clinical nurse specialist to be willing to forge new practice boundaries, perceive new ways of delivering care and take that care forward (Woods 2000). As the expert in the patient care setting, the clinical nurse specialist can envisage what constitutes high quality care and endeavour, through her leadership role, to attain that standard.

As the above demonstrates, the clinical nurse specialist role is complex, multifaceted and has to remain flexible to meet the demands of patients, nursing staff, other professionals and the employing organisation. However, further clarification of this role is required in the future; in particular with regards to the educational requirements, agreed role definition and core job description (Llahana 2005). This will allow the role to develop and positively influence patient care in both the hospital and community setting.

Community palliative care clinical nurse specialist

The community palliative care clinical nurse specialist plays a significant role in specialist palliative care in the United Kingdom, providing direct and indirect care to patients with complex or difficult to manage symptoms or needs (Skilbeck et al. 2002). These nurses are commonly known as Macmillan nurses, although not all community palliative care clinical nurse specialists carry the title 'Macmillan'. Macmillan nurse posts are initially supported by 'pump priming' monies from the charity Macmillan Cancer Support, on the understanding that their costs will subsequently be met, usually after 3 years, by the employer (Clark et al. 2002). The remit of the Macmillan nurse, when initially introduced in the 1970s, was to provide direct care to terminally ill patients; however, that role has developed and changed over the decades to that of the clinical nurse specialist (Seymour et al. 2002).

The community palliative care clinical nurse specialist is an experienced first-level registered nurse with usually a minimum of 5 years' post registration clinical experience. Prior to their appointment as clinical nurse specialists, these nurses will have had recent experience in cancer or palliative care, usually at least 2 years, and may also possess a diploma or degree in either of these subjects. Today, most of the community palliative care clinical nurse specialists will be educated to at least degree level, and many will also have completed or be undertaking a

Master's degree. A considerable number of the nurses working as community palliative care clinical nurse specialists also have a community nursing qualification, mainly in district nursing or, to a lesser extent, in health visiting. These qualifications ensure that the community palliative care clinical nurse specialist not only has knowledge of cancer and palliative care, but also an in-depth understanding of the community setting and primary health care.

The last two decades have seen an expansion in the services involved in the provision of specialist palliative care, not least the community palliative care clinical nurse specialist. These nurses are available to support patients with cancer and other life-threatening illnesses from the time they are diagnosed, and they play an important role in providing expertise in pain and symptom control and in the psychosocial support of patients and families facing advanced disease (Addington-Hall and Altmann 2000; Taylor 2004). They will intervene where there is a predefined need for which the initial referral was made, but may also discover unmet needs that have not been previously identified (Douglas et al. 2003). Intervention, after initial referral, may be by telephone contact or face-to-face visit, usually in the patient's home. The nature and frequency of ongoing contact is then determined by the clinical nurse specialist, in conjunction with the patient and carers, depending on the complex issues being addressed. Several studies have shown that their approach to care is particularly valued by patients in terms of information giving (Douglas and Venn 1999; McLoughlin 2002; Mills and Davidson 2002), increased satisfaction with care (McLoughlin 2002), increased emotional support and spiritual care (Douglas and Venn 1999). A study by Austin et al. (2000) examining perceptions of quality in palliative care found that the specialist nurse role is valued by district nurses in relation to the expertise and support the specialist service could provide; hence these specialist nurses can be described as an aid to improving the effectiveness of patient care (Douglas and Venn 1999).

It would appear therefore that referrals to community palliative care clinical nurse specialists are beneficial. However, Ahmed et al. (2004), following a systematic literature review of problems patients and professionals have in accessing specialist services, found that there is a lack of understanding amongst professionals about when to refer and to whom. According to the Scottish Executive (2001), many cancer patients and their families are being denied appropriate symptom control and support as a result of poor understanding of palliative care and the services available. This was also supported by Shipman et al. (2002) who drew attention to the variation in the way palliative care is provided within the community, and, in particular, the ways in which specialist services are utilised. It is therefore vital to ensure that district nurses, general practitioners, other members of the primary health care team and social services are aware of the range of services available, and have specific knowledge and skills and methods of accessing the community palliative care clinical nurse specialist within their own locality.

Intervention by the community palliative care clinical nurse specialist may be appropriate at any time in a patient's illness journey; however, there are a number of critical points for contact, including diagnosis, treatment and recurrence. The need for early patient referral into the specialist nursing services was noted by McLoughlin (2002), but several authors had previously examined referral patterns and found reluctance, for various reasons, on the part of some professionals to access these services (Nash 1992, 1993; Graves and Nash 1993; Skilbeck et al. 2002). Reasons given in the studies for non-referral were the lack of knowledge of the community palliative care clinical nurse specialist role, professionals indicating that they felt able and qualified to meet the needs of patients and carers, and the desire to limit the number of professionals who visited the patient. Skilbeck et al. (2002) stated in their research that, whilst the low referral rate from district nurses indicated that there may be reluctance to access these services, it may be that, simply, palliative care is now recognised as a major component of the work of the district nurse. Therefore, it is prudent to examine why and when would district nurses or other members of the primary health care team refer to the community palliative care clinical nurse specialist.

Several studies have examined the reasons for referral to the community palliative care clinical nurse specialist (Corner et al. 2002; Skilbeck et al. 2002; Bestall et al. 2004) and found similar results, emotional support for patient or carer, pain management and symptom control being the most common reasons for referral. However, Bestall et al. (2004) found that when patients had more than one symptom or problem and hence presented a case that had become complex, then referral to the community palliative care clinical nurse specialist was more likely to ensue.

A small research study conducted by Aitken (2006) set out to identify the triggers that motivate district nurses to refer patients to the community palliative care clinical nurse specialist. A number of interesting issues arose during the research, many of which supported findings in previously documented literature (Law 1997; McIlfatrick and

Curran 2000; Wright 2002; Dunne et al. 2005). The district nurses recognised that a deficit in their own clinical knowledge or skills would potentially prompt a patient's referral to the community palliative care clinical nurse specialist. This deficit was in regard to pain and symptom management, psychological support for patients and families, complex family dynamics and the information needs of patients and their carers. Interestingly, interprofessional working was also highlighted by the district nurses in Aitken's study as an area that may potentially influence referrals to the community palliative care clinical nurse specialist.

Issues regarding poor collaboration/communication with general practitioners were identified as an area of concern by some respondents and resulted in the district nurses seeking assistance from the community palliative care clinical nurse specialist to intervene in pain or symptom control. In palliative care, interprofessional working is paramount to good service provision (Hughes 2004), where general practitioners, district nurses, community palliative care clinical nurse specialists and others work together to complement and enhance the care that they provide, with communication being a key element of the interprofessional teamwork.

However, not all district nurses may be aware of when to ask the community palliative care clinical nurse specialist for intervention; Aitken's study revealed a very apparent lack of knowledge regarding the role of the specialist nurse. The findings identified that not all the district nurses were fully aware what services the community palliative care clinical nurse specialist could offer to patients, and therefore this lack of knowledge may have impaired the decision-making process regarding referrals. This may result in missed opportunities to assist patients with complex physical or psychological problems due to late referrals or, indeed, no referral to the service.

The literature reveals that reasons and timing for referral to the community palliative care clinical nurse specialist are complex; however, palliative care itself is complex and is shaped as much by organisational context as by the skills of those professionals who deliver it (Clark et al. 2002). Nurses working in palliative care need to make decisions to meet the complex physical, psychological and spiritual needs of patients and families, and this requires a knowledge of services available and recognition that supporting patients throughout their illness trajectory requires the skills of all members of the multidisciplinary team working in partnership with the patient and his or her family (Andrew and Whyte 2004).

Key Points

- Clinical nurse specialists can be defined as experts in a particular field of nursing, possessing advanced education, linking theory to practice and ensuring that nursing care is research based and of a high standard.
- The clinical nurse specialist role incorporates five areas of practice: clinical, research, consultative, education and leadership.
- The community palliative care clinical nurse specialist plays a significant role in specialist palliative care in the United Kingdom.
- These nurses are available to support patients with cancer and other life-threatening illnesses from the time they are diagnosed and play an important role in providing expertise in symptom control and in the psychosocial support of patients and their families facing advanced disease.
- Supporting patients throughout their illness trajectory requires the skills of all members of the multidisciplinary team working in partnership with the patient and his or her family.

Useful resources

Castledine G, McGee P (eds) (1998) *Advanced and Specialist Nursing Practice*. Blackwell Science, Oxford.

Clark D, Seymour J, Douglas HR, et al. (2002) Clinical Nurse Specialists in Palliative Care. Part 2: Explaining Diversity in the Organisation and Costs of Macmillan Nursing Services. *Palliative Medicine* 16 (5), 375–385.

Llahana SV (2005) *A Theoretical Framework for Clinical Specialist Nursing: An Example from Diabetes*. APS, Salisbury.

McGhee P, Castledine G (eds) (2003) *Advanced Nursing Practice*, 2nd edn. Blackwell Publishing, Oxford.

Seymour J, Clark D, Hughes P, et al. (2002) Clinical Nurse Specialists in Palliative Care. Part 3: Issues for the Macmillan Nurse Role. *Palliative Medicine* 16 (5), 386–394.

Skilbeck J, Corner J, Bath P, et al. (2002) Clinical Nurse Specialists in Palliative Care. Part 1: A Description of the Macmillan Nurse Caseload. *Palliative Medicine* 16 (4), 285–296.

References

Addington-Hall J, Altmann D (2000) Which terminally ill cancer patients in the United Kingdom receive care from community specialist palliative care nurses? *Journal of Advanced Nursing* 32 (4), 799–806.

Ahmed N, Bestall JC, Ahmedzai SH, Payne S, Clark D, Noble B (2004) Systematic review of the problems and issues of accessing specialist palliative care by patients, carers and health and social care professionals. *Palliative Medicine* 18 (6), 525–542.

Aitken A (2006) District nurses' triggers for referral of patients to the Macmillan nurse. *British Journal of Community Nursing* 11 (3), 100–107.

Andrew J, Whyte F (2004) The experiences of district nurses caring for people receiving palliative chemotherapy. *International Journal of Palliative Nursing* 10 (3), 110–118.

Armstrong P (1999) The role of the clinical nurse specialist. *Nursing Standard* 13 (16), 40–42.

Austin L, Luker K, Caress A, Hallet C (2000) Palliative care: community nurses' perceptions of quality. *Quality in Health Care* 9 (3), 151–158.

Barron AM (1989) The CNS as consultant. In: Hamric AB, Spross JA (eds) *The Clinical Nurse Specialist in Theory and Practice*, 2nd edn, pp 125–146. WB Saunders, Philadelphia.

Bestall JC, Ahmed N, Ahmedzai SH, Payne SA, Noble B, Clark D (2004) Access and referral to specialist palliative care: patients' and professionals' experiences. *International Journal of Palliative Nursing* 10 (8), 381–389.

Bousfield C (1997) A phenomenological investigation into the role of the clinical nurse specialist. *Journal of Advanced Nursing* 25 (2), 245–256.

Castledine G (2003) The development of advanced nursing practice in the UK. In: McGhee P, Castledine G (eds) *Advanced Nursing Practice*, 2nd edn, pp 8–16. Blackwell Publishing, Oxford.

Castledine G, McGee P (eds) (1998) *Advanced and Specialist Nursing Practice*. Blackwell Science, Oxford.

Clark D, Seymour J, Douglas HR, et al. (2002) Clinical nurse specialists in palliative care. Part 2: Explaining diversity in the organisation and costs of Macmillan nursing services. *Palliative Medicine* 16 (5), 375–385.

Corner J, Clark D, Normand C (2002) Evaluating the work of clinical nurse specialists in palliative care. *Palliative Medicine* 16 (4), 275–277.

Department of Health (2004) *The NHS Knowledge and Skills Framework and Related Development Review*. Department of Health, London.

Department of Health and Social Security (1972) *Report of the Committee on Nursing*. HMSO, London.

Douglas HR, Halliday D, Normand C, et al. (2003) Economic evaluation of specialist cancer and palliative nursing: Macmillan evaluation study findings. *International Journal of Palliative Nursing* 9 (10), 429–438.

Douglas J, Venn S (1999) An audit of the community Macmillan nursing service. *Journal of Community Nursing* 13 (11), 24–26, 28.

Dunne K, Sullivan K, Kernohan G (2005) Palliative care for patients with cancer: district nurses' experiences. *Journal of Advanced Nursing* 50 (4), 372–380.

Gournic JL (1989) Clinical leadership management and the CNS. In: Hamric AB, Spross JA (eds) *The Clinical Nurse Specialist in Theory and Practice*, 2nd edn, pp 227–260. WB Saunders, Philadelphia.

Graves D, Nash A (1993) Referring patients for domiciliary care. *Nursing Standard* 7 (24), 25–28.

Hamric AB, Spross JA (eds) (1989) *The Clinical Nurse Specialist in Theory and Practice*, 2nd edn. WB Saunders, Philadelphia.

Hughes L (2004) Palliative care in the community. *Primary Health Care* 14 (6), 27–31.

Koetters TL (1989) Clinical practice and direct patient care. In: Hamric AB, Spross JA (eds) *The Clinical Nurse Specialist in Theory and Practice*, 2nd edn, pp 107–123. WB Saunders, Philadelphia.

Law R (1997) The quality of district nursing care for dying patients. *Nursing Standard* 5 (12), 41–44.

Llahana SV (2005) *A Theoretical Framework for Clinical Specialist Nursing: An Example from Diabetes*. APS, Salisbury.

McGuire DB, Harwood KV (1989) The CNS as researcher. In: Hamric AB, Spross JA (eds) *The Clinical Nurse Specialist in Theory and Practice*, 2nd edn, pp 169–203. WB Saunders, Philadelphia.

McIlfatrick S, Curran C (2000) District nurses' perceptions of palliative care services: part 2. *International Journal of Palliative Nursing* 6 (1), 32–38.

McLoughlin PA (2002) Community specialist palliative care: experiences of patients and carers. *International Journal of Palliative Nursing* 8 (7), 344–353.

Miller S (1995) The clinical nurse specialist: a way forward. *Journal of Advanced Nursing* 22 (3), 494–501.

Mills M, Davidson R (2002) Cancer patients' sources of information: use and quality issues. *Psycho-Oncology* 11 (5), 371–378.

Nash A (1992) Patterns and trends in referrals to a palliative nursing service. *Journal of Advanced Nursing* 17 (4), 432–440.

Nash A (1993) Reasons for referral to a palliative nursing team. *Journal of Advanced Nursing* 18 (5), 707–713.

Priest AR (1989) The CNS as educator. In: Hamric AB, Spross JA (eds) *The Clinical Nurse Specialist in Theory and Practice*, 2nd edn, pp 147–167. WB Saunders, Philadelphia.

Reiter F (1966) The nurse clinician. *American Journal of Nursing* 66 (2), 274–280.

Reveley S, Walsh M, Crumbie A (eds) (2001) *Nurse Practitioners: Developing the Role in Hospital Settings.* Butterworth Heinemann, Oxford.

Scottish Executive Health Department (2001) *Cancer in Scotland: Action for Change.* Scottish Executive, Edinburgh.

Seymour J, Clark D, Hughes P, et al. (2002) Clinical nurse specialists in palliative care. Part 3: Issues for the Macmillan nurse role. *Palliative Medicine* 16 (5), 386–394.

Shipman C, Addington-Hall J, Barclay S, et al. (2002) How and why do GPs use specialist palliative care services? *Palliative Medicine* 16 (3), 241–246.

Skilbeck J, Corner J, Bath P, et al. (2002) Clinical nurse specialists in palliative care. Part 1: A description of the Macmillan nurse caseload. *Palliative Medicine* 16 (4), 285–296.

Taylor C (2004) Reviewing nursing support in cancer care. *Cancer Nursing Practice* 3 (3), 26–31.

United Kingdom Central Council for Nursing Midwifery and Health Visiting (1994) *Standards for Education and Practice Following Registration.* UKCC, London.

United Kingdom Central Council for Nursing Midwifery and Health Visiting (1998) *A Higher Level of Practice.* UKCC, London.

Woods LP (2000) *The Enigma of Advanced Nursing Practice.* Quay Books, Salisbury.

Wright K (2002) Caring for the terminally ill: the district nurse's perspective. *British Journal of Nursing* 11 (18), 1180–1185.

Section II
Patients

Living with a Life-Threatening Illness

Introduction

Receiving the diagnosis of cancer, or other life-threatening illness, is shocking and overwhelming (Wells 2001). Life is turned upside down and the patient faces a future of uncertainty. His or her world suddenly becomes unpredictable. Each individual will deal with the knowledge differently, but it is essential to understand the impact that the diagnosis has on the person. He/she may face months of treatments, surgery, body image changes or distressing symptoms. The community palliative care clinical nurse specialist can provide the information, advice and support needed throughout the illness trajectory, but particularly at difficult times such as diagnosis, treatment, recurrence and facing death. This chapter explores, with the help of patient scenarios, the role of the community palliative care clinical nurse specialist in providing care and support to patients with complex needs who are living with a life-threatening illness.

Diagnosis

The diagnosis of a life-threatening illness can be devastating, with many patients unable to absorb the information being given. Most individuals do not want to be told they are unwell and may resent the intrusion of this disease into their lives. Their journey may indeed have started many weeks or months previously, when they first visited their general practitioner with vague troubling symptoms. In some instances, the patient may have visited the doctor because he/she had detected a problem, such as a breast lump or bloody cough, and this will have caused uncertainty and worry about possible causes of the symptoms. The patient may have endured invasive and embarrassing tests and procedures, visits to various hospital departments, X-rays and scans, all creating considerable anxiety, before the final consultation which imparts the bad news. Like many patients, Mary, a school teacher in her 30s, visited the doctor rarely.

Case Story: Mary

Mary had found that her right knee had been swelling and giving her occasional pain. After some weeks she visited the general practitioner who prescribed analgesia and rest, not so easy for an active school teacher. Some months later Mary was still concerned as she noticed that the swelling was now present all the time and giving more pain. However, she did not go back to the general practitioner until she was having difficulty walking on the leg, due to the pain. She was immediately referred to the orthopaedic specialist and after investigation was found to have a sarcoma. Mary was devastated.

Mary rarely went to the general practitioner and did not want to 'bother them' with her painful leg. However, other patients may visit their surgery regularly and have an established trusting relationship with their general practitioner. This can then be torn apart at diagnosis; this happened with Carol, a nursing assistant in her 40s.

Case Story: Carol

Carol had been diagnosed with rheumatoid arthritis some years previously. This did not stop her from leading a very full and active life. She had a good relationship with her general practitioner and thought of her more as a friend. Carol started having back pains; she described these as different from her normal aches. The general practitioner had related the pain to her rheumatoid arthritis and had tried various new analgesics with limited success. Over a period of many months, Carol visited the doctor on numerous occasions to report the success or mainly failure of the analgesics. Her pain was now increasing in severity. The general practitioner decided that the physiotherapist may be able to offer advice on Carol's pain. Before the appointment arrived, Carol woke up one morning to find she was having difficulty walking. Carol was admitted as an emergency to the local hospital and after several bewildering days of investigations was informed she had advanced metastatic breast cancer with spinal cord compression. Carol was angry, very angry.

There will also be times when patients, knowingly or unknowingly, cause a delay in their diagnosis. Various reasons include a lack of knowledge on the part of the patient, perhaps not realising that the symptom was indicative of a serious illness; being so terrified of cancer that they do not go to the general practitioner for fear of what they may find; embarrassment about symptoms that may involve bladder, bowel or sexual function; concealment of symptoms for various reasons.

Case Story: Janet

Janet was living alone, having been divorced several years before. She had an ongoing long-term condition for which she attended the general practitioner regularly. One day, during a routine consultation, she asked the female general practitioner if she would look at a wound on her chest wall. Janet had an extensive breast cancer covering her left chest wall. She later informed the community palliative care clinical nurse specialist that it had been present for many years, growing from an initial small break to the extensive lesion she now had. She reported always knowing what it was and that it was difficulties with dressing the wound that had forced her to ask for assistance. Janet admitted she had initially been afraid of the lesion, but had become accepting of its presence, and possible outcome, over the years.

As illustrated, reactions to a life-threatening diagnosis can be different. However, there are some patients, as in the case of Sarah, who find it almost a relief to be told their diagnosis. They may have suspected for some time that they have a serious or life-threatening illness, and to finally have the diagnosis can help them deal with their anxiety and uncertainty.

Case Story: Sarah

Sarah, a single lady in her 60s, was very active in her local community. She had started to notice some minor difficulties in her speech and choking occasionally when eating. Sarah was concerned about this, but did not go to the general practitioner until her friend urged her to seek help. Sarah was eventually diagnosed with motor neurone disease. This came as a relief to Sarah, as she knew how to deal with

---

Case Story: Sarah (*continued*)

this diagnosis; her father and sister had died from the illness. She had feared that she may have had cancer of the throat and this had caused her more anxiety than the reality of motor neurone disease.

Emotional impact of diagnosis

When someone is diagnosed with cancer or some other life-threatening illness, the most common response is shock (Brennan 2004). Initially they may describe a feeling of numbness, where the reality of the situation has yet to be absorbed. This may last for hours, days or in some cases for weeks. Naturally this is a time of emotional turmoil; early reactions may be anger, guilt, anxiety or sadness (Palmer and Howarth 2005). How each patient copes with these emotions is a highly individual matter (Cooper 1993). As time goes on, the reality of the situation becomes apparent and the patient may become distressed and emotionally vulnerable (Barraclough 1999). As the information is assimilated, it is important to allow the patient the opportunity to talk about his or her complex feelings. A skilled professional, such as the community palliative care clinical nurse specialist, may be able to encourage patients to disclose their initial worries or fears, to give them time to make sense of the news that has just been delivered.

As demonstrated above, each individual responds differently, but, in common, everyone needs time and the opportunity to express emotions. An understanding of the variety of reactions to illness will help the community palliative care clinical nurse specialist to respond in a sensitive and timely manner. Mary was completely unaware that her knee problem may be the result of anything serious and was totally devastated. She found it difficult to talk initially and needed space for her own thoughts. Carol was very angry; she expressed her anger through shouting and tears. She worried about her family and how they would cope, not just in the future, but whilst she was in hospital having treatment. Janet had a mixture of emotions ranging from guilt, due to her concealment of the lesion, to relief, because at last she was receiving help to deal with her cancer. Sarah was very quiet and accepting of her diagnosis. However, she was keen to look ahead to practical issues, as she was well aware of the debility that the illness would bring. It is not difficult to see that the diagnosis of cancer or other life-threatening illness can be devastating, indeed one of the most stressful times for patients (Brennan 2004), but the response can also be affected by how the news is delivered.

Receiving bad news

Most patients are given the news of their diagnosis from a doctor. This interview can have a profound effect on their initial reaction to the news and subsequent ability to deal with their illness. Despite many texts on breaking bad news, it is still carried out very poorly by some professionals.

Case Story: Tom

Tom had been retired for some years. He noticed that he had started to gain some weight around his abdomen, but assumed it was due to his reduced physical activity. However, he decided to visit his general practitioner for some advice on weight control. He was very surprised when the general practitioner informed him that he had fluid gathering on his abdomen and wanted him admitted to hospital for investigation. A few days later, on a Friday afternoon, a doctor whom Tom had not seen previously, approached his bed and informed him that he had his test results. Without pulling the screens, to allow for privacy, the doctor informed Tom that he had cancer and that there would be no treatment. Tom was shocked. He was informed that he would be discharged that day, as no more could be done for him. Tom had been alone; his wife was not due to visit until the evening. He contacted a friend and arranged a lift home. He could not bring himself to speak to his wife on the telephone. When he did get home he had to relay the information to his wife. It was Friday evening, the local surgery was closed and they had to cope with this news on their own all weekend. On the Monday morning his wife contacted the local surgery and the general practitioner visited, but he had no information from the hospital and therefore could not answer any of their questions. The couple were angry and upset and at every opportunity Tom relayed this scenario to all the health professionals who subsequently visited the house. This anger stayed with Tom during the remaining few weeks of his life.

Communicating a diagnosis of a life-threatening illness, such as cancer, is difficult for the health professional as well as for the patient who is receiving the news (Wells 2001). This work never becomes easy and will always be stressful for the health professional. However, breaking bad news is an important part of the role of professionals and requires experience and expertise (Buckman 1995). They must take into consideration that the bad news about to be given will dramatically and unpleasantly alter the patient's life (Twycross 1997).

All individuals experience losses throughout their lives, but when bad news is given, the way it is delivered can assist or prevent patients in working through their grieving process (Young 2001). Depending on how this news is conveyed, it may leave the patient feeling not only angry but also resentful towards the doctor. The shock, fear and devastation of hearing bad news may mean that information is just not being absorbed. Unfortunately, so many of these encounters take place in a busy outpatient clinic and patients have limited time to assimilate the information and ask appropriate questions before they are ushered out of the room. This leaves the patient not only shocked, particularly if the diagnosis had not been suspected, but also unable to remember most of the consultation beyond the word *cancer*. Therefore, they have no clear understanding of treatment options, likely outcomes, or indeed when they are to be seen again.

For some patients, the diagnosis itself may leave them bewildered; they may never have heard about the disease the doctor is talking about, for example motor neurone disease. The diagnosis is bound to raise further questions, perhaps in relation to treatments, prognosis or more practical issues, for example transport to and from the hospital for treatments. In situations of stress, such as receiving bad news, research has shown that short-term memory and concentration become poor and people have difficulty absorbing new information (Brennan 2004). As a result, there may be an urgent need for further advice and rechecking of information already given, as well as supportive care to address the psychological distress associated with the diagnosis.

Emotional and practical support

In order to assist these patients with their emotional distress a referral may be made to the community palliative care clinical nurse specialist from other members of the primary health care team or hospital oncology unit. The community palliative care clinical nurse specialist is available to give further information and also emotional and practical support to these patients with complex needs, from the time of their diagnosis. It will be necessary to acknowledge how difficult it must be for patients, encourage them to talk, clarify their understanding of the situation and also to give information that is relevant and when the patient is ready to accept it. What is communicated must be appropriate and in a language that the patient understands. However, patients may find it difficult to talk about their diagnosis and their emotions; they may find it awkward or embarrassing trying to communicate, not only with their family and friends, but also with the health professionals (Buckman 1995). Within many families, individuals are not always accustomed to disclosing and talking about their innermost feelings. This requires the community palliative care clinical nurse specialist to be sensitive to patients' needs and encourage them to express their fears and concerns when they feel able and comfortable to discuss these delicate issues.

Case Story: Sandy

Sandy was 66 years of age and a retired shipyard worker. He had just been diagnosed with mesothelioma. He had heard about this illness at work, as one of his workmates had died from the disease in the previous year. Sandy's wife was worried; Sandy had never been a communicative man and refused to talk about the illness or his feelings. The community palliative care clinical nurse specialist was asked to visit to assist Sandy's wife with her complex emotions and the lack of dialogue between the couple. Sandy enjoyed working in his garden. The community palliative care clinical nurse specialist realised the garden was where Sandy felt comfortable. Very gradually, after visits to his wife, the nurse would spend a few minutes in the garden discussing the flowers, the plants, etc. with Sandy. Eventually Sandy started to discuss his fatigue and the impact this was having on his ability to maintain his garden. Very gradually Sandy started to express his emotions; it was only ever for a few minutes at a time but it was at Sandy's pace. He started to ask questions and, after several visits, his wife eventually joined Sandy and the nurse in the garden. It had been important to gain Sandy's trust and to keep the dialogue within safe boundaries. It allowed Sandy to gradually discuss the issues that were important to him, and to ask questions when he was ready.

If patients are to be involved in decisions about their care and treatment, they require knowledge about their diagnosis, prognosis, treatment options and potential side-effects (Doyle and Jeffrey 2000). The community palliative care clinical nurse specialist is able to spend time explaining medical terminology, discussing the various tests and results, helping patients to feel more reassured about their future treatments, answering questions and listening to their concerns and fears. Many patients will feel more relaxed in their own homes, with the familiar surroundings giving a sense of security. This may allow patients to absorb more material and also to ask more questions about their illness. It also allows an opportunity to address issues of a more practical nature which may be troubling the patient. Listening is probably the most important skill at this time (Palmer and Howarth 2005). Actively listening to patients may do much to allay their fears and allow them to express their emotions; the community palliative care clinical nurse specialist has the expertise and skills to provide the specialist care needed at this time.

According to Skilbeck and Payne (2004), communication is one of the most important aspects of nursing care in improving outcomes for patients with a life-threatening illness, particularly those experiencing psychological and emotional distress. Good communication skills help to establish a trusting relationship between the patient and the professional, allowing uncertainties to be confronted and explored (Doyle and Jeffrey 2000). Community palliative care clinical nurse specialists are experienced nurses with considerable communication skills; their careful assessment of the patient allows for an honest and sensitive exchange, where they can follow the patient's agenda and explore the patient's fears and emotions. The communication skills of the community palliative care clinical nurse specialist are invaluable in assisting patients along their cancer journey. However, it should be noted that not all patients with a life-threatening illness will be seen or want to be seen by a community palliative care clinical nurse specialist. For many patients the support given by the other members of the experienced primary health care team will suffice their needs. Referrals are made to the community palliative care clinical nurse specialist for those patients who have complex needs.

No matter how experienced the health professional, talking to patients can be challenging (Jeffrey 1998) and at times the professional can get it wrong. As previously mentioned, Tom had a very bad experience when receiving his diagnosis. He remained angry throughout his illness; he stated that under no circumstances would he go back into hospital. The role of the community palliative care clinical nurse specialist was therefore to acknowledge Tom's anger, listen to his concerns, explain possible scenarios resulting from his deteriorating condition and ensure he was fully informed when making his decision. He required constant reassurance that the primary health care team was fully aware of his wishes and that he would be allowed to die at home. The community palliative care clinical nurse specialist visited Tom on many occasions; he reported finding the visits beneficial and helped him to gain confidence in remaining at home throughout his cancer journey.

Following their diagnosis, all patients will have considerable concerns about their illness, possible treatments, their prognosis and future life (Brennan 2004). For those diagnosed with cancer, they will find that the illness and its treatment (even when the aim is palliative) is complex and the journey may be difficult and stressful. Unfortunately, patients with a cancer diagnosis are confronted with many ongoing stressors, rather than a single time-limited crisis (Groenwald et al. 1997).

Treatment

After the initial shock of the diagnosis, the patient has to try to assimilate all the information he/she has been given regarding possible treatments. Many patients already have some prior knowledge of cancer treatments. However, this knowledge may be as a result of television coverage, magazine or newspaper articles or indeed from family, friends or a neighbour. Sadly, many tales are told that do not always give truthful or realistic accounts and leave the patient feeling frightened and confused.

Case Story: Joyce

Joyce was a hard-working lady in her 60s who had been diagnosed with lung cancer. Her disease had produced a metastatic adrenal mass and her oncologist advised chemotherapy. Joyce declined the treatment. Some years previously, Joyce's friend had died from cancer. Joyce's recollection was of her friend dying with no hair, considerably overweight, confused and unable to care for herself. Her friend's husband blamed the chemotherapy for his wife's death. Joyce was therefore determined not to accept the treatment as she was afraid the chemotherapy would bring about her own death in a similar fashion.

Joyce required accurate information regarding possible treatment and a referral was made to the community palliative care clinical nurse specialist, from the oncologist, to visit Joyce at home. This allowed her an opportunity to discuss her fears and concerns within the security of her own surroundings. It is important to be honest with the information, so that the patient is not falsely reassured that a treatment, such as chemotherapy, is relatively mild when it may cause side-effects and hence the patient becomes distrustful of the health professionals (Faulkner and Maguire 1994). Patients require to know what side-effects are likely, how long they may last and what can be done to alleviate them (Faull and Barton 1998). Most patients look positively towards treatment because they hope it may overcome or control their disease (Barraclough 1999); however, at the same time they regard it with apprehension because of the side-effects. There is nothing pleasant about today's cancer treatments and patients are quite rightly fearful of them.

Case Story: Margaret

Margaret had developed ovarian cancer in her 50s. She was to have six cycles of intravenous chemotherapy at three-weekly intervals. Pain control had been a problem, but after adjustment of her medication she reported an improvement. Prior to her first cycle of treatment she telephoned the district nursing service on many occasions over 2–3 days, requesting input for a variety of minor problems. This happened again on the days preceding her second cycle of treatment. The nurses were aware that Margaret seemed very anxious during these visits. A referral was made to the community palliative care clinical nurse specialist for assistance. Margaret was initially reluctant to talk about her feelings, but gradually began to express her fear of the chemotherapy. She reported the anguish of 'poison' going through her veins. Her fear of the treatment was even greater than her fear of the cancer. Margaret was encouraged to express these fears and, having acknowledged them, found that she was able to look at the more positive aspects of what the chemotherapy was doing to her cancer. She managed to complete the remaining four cycles of treatment.

Information needs

If patients are to participate in decisions about their treatment, they need to have a clear idea of the goal of care (Jeffrey 2000). Are the aims of treatment curative or palliative; perhaps to extend survival time, or to alleviate symptoms; or is it being given because of an immediate problem, such as spinal cord compression? The role of the community palliative care clinical nurse specialist allows time to discuss these issues with patients and to provide information regarding the aims of treatment and what will happen during treatment. The community palliative care clinical nurse specialist, through her links with the oncology consultants, is able to gather the appropriate information and relay this to the patient. Patients will appreciate assistance in translating the medical jargon which they may not understand, and, at times, the community palliative care clinical nurse specialist may be acting as an advocate for patients to ensure that their voice and opinions are considered when treatment decisions are being made by the medical professional (Akkerman 1998).

Case Story: Fred

Fred was a real character who always enjoyed a good laugh and going out socialising. He had been having problems with shortness of breath for some time and had eventually been persuaded to go to the general practitioner. He was diagnosed with lung cancer and bone metastases. He had been to see the oncologist who had offered palliative radiotherapy. Fred was having none of these modern treatments. The community palliative care clinical nurse specialist was asked to visit Fred and assess his comprehension of the situation and also to give him information about the proposed treatment. Fred expressed his complete lack of understanding about it all, although he was fully aware that he was going to die from the lung cancer. He listened whilst the nurse explained the situation, and then thanked her for discussing it in a way he could understand. However, he asked the community palliative care clinical nurse specialist to inform the oncologist he had not changed his mind about treatment and to make it clear that he did not want any more hospital appointments, but would take each day as it came. The role of the community palliative care clinical nurse specialist was to act as Fred's advocate and ensure his wishes were relayed to the oncologist and the other members of the health care team.

When dealing with cancer, the treatment is multifaceted, with one treatment mode or perhaps combinations being used depending on the patient's cancer, stage of disease, age, co-morbidity, general frailty, etc. Patients may just want to get started with their treatment, believing that any delay may jeopardise their survival; however, they do need time to adjust to their diagnosis, obtain all the relevant information, make decisions regarding treatment and fully discuss issues with their oncologist. Treatment should be started as soon as possible, but delays of a few weeks probably make little difference to the final outcome of the cancer (Barraclough 1999); however, this needs to be conveyed to the anxious patient. The main treatments for cancer comprise surgery, chemotherapy or radiotherapy, although other treatments such as immunotherapy or hormone treatment, for example, may be used. Mixed in with this cocktail of treatments is also the need for symptom control and management of the patient's emotional distress (Blows 2005).

After discussion with the patient, a referral may be passed onto the community palliative care clinical nurse specialist from the oncologist or general practitioner to assist the patient in understanding the proposed treatment and to offer emotional support during this distressing time. The role of the community palliative care clinical nurse specialist is to assist patients to understand what has been discussed with their doctors, in regard to the treatment on offer, its potential benefits in relation to their disease, length of treatment and side-effects. Explanation can be given to patients in their own home, where they may be able to ask more questions and absorb more of the details of what is being communicated. This follow-up interview also enables questions to be answered that may have arisen in the interval between the patient seeing the hospital consultant and the nurse visiting.

The community palliative care clinical nurse specialist also has to take into account, when communicating information, that the patient may be feeling unwell from a variety of symptoms and having difficulty in concentrating on new information. A nursing assessment needs to be undertaken to determine problematic symptoms and, following discussion with the general practitioner, the appropriate action taken. Although patients seen by the community palliative care clinical nurse specialist have in common the diagnosis of a life-threatening illness, many of the problems with which they struggle depend on the stage and type of disease. Common symptoms that patients may be experiencing are pain, nausea, fatigue and emotional distress. Cancer patients, in particular, may find these symptoms almost overwhelming (Buckman 1995). Advice, information and strategies for dealing with symptoms will be discussed with the patient, and in collaboration with the general practitioner or palliative medicine consultant, medication prescribed appropriately and its effects monitored by the community palliative care clinical nurse specialist or primary health care team.

As mentioned above, standard treatments for cancer fall into three main types: surgery, radiotherapy and chemotherapy. Most of the patients who are seen by the community palliative care clinical nurse specialist will be having palliative treatment. The most obvious aim of palliation is to improve quality of life and relieve tumour-related symptoms (Hoskin and Makin 2003). These treatments may change the course of the disease, leading to either longer survival or a reduction in symptoms, and in some cases to both (Napier and Srinivasan 2002), but will not alter the inevitable outcome of the disease. The decision to initiate palliative therapies is often complex, as the possible benefits must be balanced against any side-effects. However, some decisions are easier to make, such as radiotherapy to painful bone metastases or surgery to relieve a bowel obstruction. Chemotherapy also has a significant role in palliation; however, patients receiving this therapy are those most likely to respond; this will be determined by taking into account the tumour type, previous treatments, disease-free interval and patient performance status (Napier and Srinivasan 2002).

Chemotherapy

The role of the community palliative care clinical nurse specialist is to give information to patients as requested and assist them to understand the complex treatments they are going to receive. This requires the community palliative care clinical nurse specialist to have a considerable in-depth knowledge of cancer treatments and their side-effects. Chemotherapy means drug treatment and is usually administered orally or intravenously, depending on the drugs used, and is divided into a number of doses, given in regular cycles and may continue for several months. The patients will be given a full explanation regarding their chemotherapy from the consultant in the clinic, or from the nurses in the chemotherapy ward. However, as often happens, some are unable to recall the information when they go home.

The general practitioner may ask for the community palliative care clinical nurse specialist to assist patients with their information needs. Since the prospect of chemotherapy is likely to raise fears and concerns, the community palliative care clinical nurse specialist should start by exploring the patient's understanding of the treatment (Brennan 2004). Patients require explanation regarding the drugs, how they will be administered and when they will be given. It is important for patients to know if the drugs are to be given as an outpatient in the day ward or if they will require hospitalisation. Because chemotherapy is a systemic therapy, the drugs will kill healthy dividing cells as well as cancer cells, and this can be associated with some severe unwanted side-effects (Barraclough 1999). The side-effects will vary depending on the drugs the patient is to receive, but common side-effects are nausea and vomiting, diarrhoea, sore mouth, hair loss, tiredness and bone marrow depression. Because of the toxic effects of chemotherapy on the bone marrow, a reduction in the number of red blood cells, white blood cells and platelets can occur. The blood counts reach their lowest point 7–14 days after treatment and during this time patients are at risk of infection and haemorrhagic complications. These complications can be life-threatening and patients need appropriate information regarding these side effects.

Case Story: Marion

Marion had metastatic lung cancer. She suffered from repeated chest infections during her illness and usually required a course of oral antibiotics to clear the infection. She was having palliative chemotherapy to try to alleviate symptoms of her disease. About 8 days after her chemotherapy (on a Friday) she noticed she was expectorating green sputum. She was aware that she should report infections, but thought she would wait until after the weekend to contact her general practitioner. Apart from fatigue, she had no other symptoms. On the Sunday her condition changed markedly, her husband contacted the out-of-hours service and she was admitted to hospital. Marion was seriously unwell. Her husband was shocked at how quickly his wife had deteriorated and that her condition was now life-threatening.

Marion had been well informed about the potential risks of infection, but, sadly, even with full explanation from the chemotherapy nurses and written information, had still not appreciated the need for immediate action should she develop signs of infection. It is not always possible to know what information is being absorbed when communicating with patients and if it is being fully understood; unfortunately written material may never be read. If the patient is particularly anxious or the staff in the chemotherapy room are concerned about the level of information retention and the patient's understanding of the treatment, then a referral can be made to the community palliative care clinical nurse specialist for assistance. The community palliative care clinical nurse specialist can visit and clarify the facts again with the patient in his/her own home, and also explain about the written information. Giving the information again to the patient may potentially reduce the likelihood of a life-threatening situation arising.

Other patients may have read all the information, but their recollection of friends or family having treatment is paramount in their minds and creating anxiety.

Case Story: Jess

Jess, a married lady in her 70s, was diagnosed with metastatic bowel cancer. She was to have six cycles of chemotherapy. She had read all the literature regarding her treatment, but was concerned when it stated that she may have nausea. She was not due to see her oncologist again for 2 weeks and therefore contacted the community palliative care clinical nurse specialist for advice. Her only experience of cancer was when a friend died some years before. She recalled that her friend had had some form of treatment and had vomited a lot afterwards. She reported being worried that she may vomit excessively and would have to rely on her husband for assistance. This was causing her considerable anxiety.

Nausea and vomiting are still the most common and unwanted side-effects of chemotherapy; however, significant progress has been made in the treatment of this problem with the range of modern anti-emetic drugs now available. It also has to be explained to patients that not all the chemotherapy drugs have the same degree of side-effects and that patients are individual in their reactions to the treatment. Jess was reassured and relieved to be informed by the community palliative care clinical nurse specialist that the chemotherapy regime she was to be given caused only very mild nausea and that she would be supplied with anti-emetics to take at home if required. This reassurance involved only a short telephone call, but brought immense relief to the patient.

The importance of clear information regarding therapies such as chemotherapy and also radiotherapy cannot be overstated. The most common source of anxiety regarding the treatments comes from fear of the unknown (Brennan 2004). Information to the patient should always start with the patient's pre-existing knowledge of the proposed treatment. As with chemotherapy, there is also fear about radiotherapy.

Radiotherapy

Radiotherapy plays a significant role in the treatment of the most common cancers and also contributes to the palliation of metastases, particularly those in the bone and brain (Coyler 2003). Radiotherapy is most commonly delivered using a linear accelerator that produces high-energy X-ray beams. It involves the targeted delivery of radiation to the malignant growth. Most radiotherapy is pre-planned and given as an outpatient; the treatment will last for only a few minutes and have no accompanying symptoms at the time of delivery. However, an emergency situation may occur when a patient has to be treated urgently, for example spinal cord compression or superior vena cava obstruction.

Over 50% of all radiotherapy given in the United Kingdom is with palliative intent (Hoskin and Makin 2003). As previously mentioned, most treatment is given as an outpatient and therefore the patient may have to travel a considerable distance each day for a treatment lasting only a few minutes. The treatment is delivered in a room with no familiar trappings and the patient will be alone under a large and intimidating machine. The actual treatment process causes no pain; indeed there is nothing to feel at all whilst the treatment is being delivered (Barraclough 1999). However, some patients do find that maintaining a particular position to have the treatment may be uncomfortable.

Radiotherapy is a local treatment and its effects are limited to the site where the treatment is being targeted. However, radiotherapy side-effects can have considerable consequences, both physically and psychologically, and can cause debilitating chronic problems with reduced quality of life (Faithful 2001). Palliative treatment may be given for bone pain, pathological fractures, spinal cord compression, control of haemorrhage, bronchial obstruction, dysphagia, cerebral metastases or to help dry fungating lesions on the skin (Hoskin and Makin 2003). Although palliative radiotherapy is given in such a way as to minimise side-effects, these may still occur. The nature and severity of side-effects depend on the dose given and the part of the body being treated.

Case Story: Jimmy

Jimmy was only in his 50s when diagnosed with advanced oesophageal cancer. His only complaint was difficulty swallowing some solids. He was given a palliative course of radiotherapy to try to help with his swallowing. After the treatment was complete, he complained of chest pain and he reported his swallowing as considerably worse. He also complained of overwhelming tiredness. He felt that the treatment had not only been a waste of time, but also made his symptoms unbearable. He discussed these issues with the community palliative care clinical nurse specialist who reassured him that the symptoms he was experiencing were side-effects from his treatment. Appropriate symptom control and dietary advice were given and after a few weeks his pain had completely resolved and he was managing to eat most foods.

Most acute toxicity from radiotherapy is self-limiting and simply needs supportive treatment for a short period (Hoskin and Makin 2003). Where difficulties are anticipated, the radiotherapy department nurse or oncologist may refer the patient to the community palliative care clinical nurse specialist to give reassurance and advice, monitor and ensure adequate symptom control until the side-effects resolve. Adverse effects of treatment can be very debilitating and will impact on the patient's quality of life. Fatigue is recognised as a common side-effect of radiotherapy, which not only occurs during treatment but also continues for some time after the radiotherapy has ended (Faithfull 2001) and can have a negative effect on quality of life. Unfortunately side-effects tend to accumulate as treatment progresses and can be at their peak a week or two after treatment finishes. It is therefore important to explain this to patients before the commencement of treatment and make them aware that support will be available within the community afterwards to deal with symptoms that may arise. However, some patients have minimal side-effects and notice a benefit from their treatment within a short time.

Case Story: Jack

Jack had lung cancer, and was having increasing pain in his left ribs. This man, in his 80s, was having progressive difficulty with breathlessness and the pain from his ribs was felt to be contributing to his problem. He had tried increasing his analgesia with no effect, other than to make him increasingly dizzy and drowsy. His oncologist decided to give him a single fraction of palliative radiotherapy to his ribs. Jack was very sceptical that the treatment would be of benefit and the thought of the long journey to the cancer centre made him reluctant to go. A visit from the community palliative care clinical nurse specialist allowed Jack to discuss his concerns. He agreed to 'give it a go'. The treatment was very successful and allowed Jack to get out into his garden again.

Radiotherapy patients firstly need information about how the treatment works and what side-effects they may expect. The daily travelling to the hospital may prove challenging for patients, particularly if they are feeling unwell. Appropriate symptom control and provision of transport can help to alleviate the situation for the patient. Support in the community is essential for these patients, particularly after treatment has finished, when side-effects may be troublesome. Supportive care is the key element in the management of radiation side-effects and can be described as the provision of information, counselling, social support and side-effects management (Faithful 2001). Contact with the community clinical nurse specialist can assist these patients with their symptoms, give reassurance and act as a listener to their concerns. Radiotherapy is only one element of the patient's cancer journey and although treatment may have finished, the patient will require ongoing care and support from the primary health care team.

Surgery

Many of the patients who come into contact with the community palliative care clinical nurse specialist will also have undergone surgery of some description, as part of their cancer treatment. Radical surgery is probably the most effective treatment in cancer management. However, palliative surgery also plays a part in symptom relief; for example, internal fixation of a pathological fracture or to relieve an oesophageal or bowel obstruction. These procedures will have no impact on the course of the disease itself, but may bring about considerable symptom relief, therefore improving quality of life. As identified previously, patients require information about the surgery, what the operation will involve and the projected time scale for recovery. Many of the surgical procedures may be fairly minor in terms of surgical time involved, but risks versus benefits must be considered. Patients are understandably anxious about surgery and need reassurance and an opportunity to express their fears and concerns. In addition to providing information, the community palliative care clinical nurse specialist can also respond to the concerns of the patient, correcting misconceptions, and assist the patient to discuss his or her worries (Brennan 2004).

Case Story: Dorothy

Dorothy had advanced oesophageal cancer and desperately wanted to spend her last Christmas meal with her family and her grandchildren.

She was having increasing difficulty swallowing even a semi-solid diet and felt that Christmas would be miserable if she could not join the family at the festive table. Her oncologist suggested a dilatation of her oesophagus and insertion of an oesophageal stent. Dorothy was uncertain if she had the strength for surgery, but after explanation of the procedure, agreed to go ahead. She had to stay in hospital for 4 days, but found that her semi-solid diet was going down well and she regained some enjoyment in eating. She had a very emotional Christmas, but achieved her goal of sitting at the table with all her family around her and managed to eat and enjoy some of the festive fare.

The community palliative care clinical nurse specialist, after discussion with the general practitioner, had referred Dorothy back to the oncologist when her swallowing deteriorated. She required not only information on the planned procedure, but also time to express her fears about the surgery. This surgical procedure achieved a very successful outcome, with the patient achieving a major goal in her cancer journey.

Ongoing support

After treatment, whether it is radiotherapy, chemotherapy or surgery, etc., the patient will require ongoing support for weeks, months or in some cases years. The follow-up will usually be with the oncologist, but increasingly the general practitioner and the primary health care team are being relied upon to monitor the patient and refer back to the oncologist if required. It is likely that in the future the community palliative care clinical nurse specialist will play an increasing role in managing the follow-up of patients, in tandem with the general practitioner (Corner and Kelly 2001). This may be reassuring for patients, but visits to the doctor's surgery or home visits by the primary health care team and even the community palliative care clinical nurse specialist may be seen as a constant reminder of the illness and an intrusion into the patient's daily life. Patients may also become very anxious prior to medical/nursing appointments or visits, whether at the hospital, surgery or in their own homes, as discussions may reveal new symptoms that suggest progression of their disease. After treatment, fear of the cancer returning or progressing means that it is difficult for patients to return to 'normal', and contact with their health care team may be frequent as the patient looks for reassurance and support. It is important for the professionals to achieve a balance, whereby patients feel well supported and know where to get help, but also are allowed to continue living with their cancer or other life-threatening illness and enjoy some semblance of 'normality' in their lives.

When treatment finishes, whether curative or palliative, patients may feel that their 'security' has ended. They may have a sense that nothing is actually happening at present to stop their cancer. This can be a difficult time for patients and they need support and reassurance that their symptoms and cancer are being monitored. Some patients may find it difficult to live with the uncertainty that comes with their disease and need the opportunity to discuss their concerns and fears. The community palliative care clinical nurse specialist can negotiate with patients appropriate contacts, whether by telephone or visiting, to support them with their ongoing complex emotional needs during this difficult time. The threat of physical deterioration is ever present and patients who experience a recurrence of their cancer report that the news can cause greater shock and devastation than the original diagnosis.

Recurrence

Until fairly recently the recurrence of cancer was associated with terminal illness and death (Johnson and Gross 1998). However, the developments in cancer technology have resulted in more treatments being available to patients, even those whose cancer is quite advanced. Medical interventions, however, should always aim to increase not only quantity but also quality of life (Carr et al. 2001). The prospect of more treatment can in itself create anxieties for patients, particularly if they are feeling unwell and experiencing distressing symptoms. Along with the anxiety that cancer recurrence brings, the patient may have feelings of anger, injustice, fear and a sense of overwhelming loss. Many patients report that the news of recurrence is more difficult to cope with than the original diagnosis. Patients will require considerable support at this time and referral to the community palliative care clinical nurse specialist, from the primary health care team or oncologist, will allow them the opportunity to express their complex emotions, gather relevant information regarding their disease and discuss their future care needs.

Recurrence can be especially distressing for the cancer patient who believed that he/she had been cured or would survive for a number of years (Faulkner and Maguire 1994). The future for these patients now looks even more uncertain, and for some this is the inevitable outcome they have been dreading (Brennan 2004).

Case Story: Margo

Margo, a young woman in her 40s, had been diagnosed with lung cancer and had a pneumonectomy. This was followed by chemotherapy. She made a good recovery and returned to work within 8 months. She was very active and had once again started going to the gym regularly. However, her father had died from cancer and she always feared one day it might return. One weekend, 2 years after her original diagnosis, she had a seizure and was admitted to hospital where she was found to have cerebral metastases. Margo was devastated at the recurrence. She felt all the previous treatment had been in vain.

The role of the community palliative care clinical specialist is multifaceted and flexibility is required to not only deal with support and information giving, but also to facilitate patients in their emotional journey from curative treatments to palliative care. For many, the return of the illness raises fears that the cancer will now be fatal (Johnson and Gross 1998) and patients face the uncertainty of when or how death will occur.

Case Story: William

William had undergone surgery for colo-rectal cancer at the age of 58. He had always been a very sociable gentleman and belonged to many clubs, etc. He coped well with his diagnosis and had been able to 'get on with his life'. He developed some chest pain 3 years after his surgery and was found to have localised lung metastases. He again had surgery, this time to remove a lobe of his left lung. He again picked up and rejoined the activities in his social clubs. After another 18 months he started experiencing episodes of breathlessness. Once again William was found to have lung metastases, but in the right lung and quite extensive. William found this recurrence very hard. He now knew that the prognosis was poor and started having panic attacks. He had nightmares about dying and the process of dying. He believed that his death could happen suddenly and therefore he would not allow his partner to go out of the house without him. His anxiety made daily life very difficult for himself and his partner.

The community palliative care clinical nurse specialist was asked, by the district nurse, to visit this patient to assess his anxiety and explore his fears and emotions. Gradually, with the help of anxiety workshops, his symptoms started to improve and he began to sleep undisturbed at night. His breathlessness became more manageable and he experienced fewer panic attacks. The community palliative care clinical nurse specialist was able to give considerable time to this patient, a commodity that other members of the primary health care team may struggle to find in their daily schedules.

The psychological impact of recurrent disease on the patient can be exacerbated by an increase in symptoms, particularly fatigue, weakness and pain (Wells 2001). It is also important to establish what *meaning* the patient attributes to the symptoms and how the patient envisages the symptoms progressing (Davy and Ellis 2000). William, as discussed above, related his breathlessness to death, and the community palliative care clinical nurse specialist had to assess both his physical symptoms and his emotional state. It is important for patients to understand that one cannot be improved without the other being addressed.

Having to face the possibility of more active treatment is difficult for some patients. However, this time the patient is more likely to know what to expect, and, for many patients, facing more radiotherapy or chemotherapy can be devastating. They will require information about the palliative treatment on offer, its side-effects and expected outcomes. The benefits from palliative treatment have to be balanced against the side-effects, frequency of attendance at the hospital, recovery time and rehabilitation, remembering that time is limited for these patients (Hoskin and Makin 2003). For some patients, the thought of more treatment and its inevitable side-effects are overwhelming and they decline to go through it all again. Many believe that the limited time left to them might be easier to tolerate without treatment and its side-effects, allowing them to spend quality time at home (Faulkner and Maguire 1994).

Case Story: Rose

Rose was diagnosed with recurrent lung cancer a few weeks before Christmas. When offered chemotherapy, she asked the oncologist for time to talk about it with her family and think through her decision. She had nursed her husband through chemotherapy for recurrent bowel cancer and was well aware of the side-effects and emotional distress it brings. She asked her general practitioner for a visit from the community palliative care clinical nurse specialist. Rose had two young grandsons and her wish was to be with them for her last Christmas and not for the children to see her being sick and unwell. She was given the information she requested about the treatment and also allowed to discuss her anxieties and fears. Rose opted to have no treatment and indeed cancelled her subsequent contact with the oncologist. After the decision had been made to decline treatment, Rose became less anxious and enjoyed the company of her family at every opportunity.

Patients are very individual in their response to the diagnosis of recurrent cancer and, as seen above, Rose wanted to spend quality time with her family.

Case Story: Annie

Annie had no close family. She had been diagnosed with bowel cancer some years before and had undergone surgery and chemotherapy. She had recovered well and had not told her friends at that time the diagnosis, believing that there was no need for anyone to know. She had recently moved into a sheltered housing complex and had many new neighbours and friends. When an episode of diarrhoea would not clear, she had investigations which revealed advanced recurrent bowel cancer. She wanted life to continue as 'normal' for as long as possible, for whatever time she had left. She did not want her friends and neighbours to know her current diagnosis. She was supported in her decision by the community palliative care clinical nurse specialist and the primary health care team. She died quietly in the local cottage hospital with only the health professionals aware of the cause of death.

Accurate information is essential to allow patients to make informed decisions regarding treatments and feel confident in the options they choose. The community palliative care clinical nurse specialist can listen to the patient's concerns, and give advice, support and reassurance that the health care team will always be supportive, no matter what the future holds.

Facing death

Patients who are beginning the last phase of their illness and for whom life expectancy is now very limited have particular health needs (Woof et al. 1998). When told that their disease is no longer responding to treatment and is now incurable, they will once again experience emotional distress such as shock and disbelief. Feelings such as anger, anxiety, guilt and depression may also manifest themselves and they will require considerable psychological support to cope with the turmoil they may be experiencing. Painful feelings and difficult decisions may have to be addressed and for many patients it is a time when unresolved problems may resurface (Lee 2002). There are also many losses for the patient to cope with, such as the loss of future hopes and dreams (Lloyd-Williams 2004).

The support of these patients requires teamwork; the resources of the primary health care team and the community palliative care clinical nurse specialist working collaboratively, to ease the patient's journey. The choice of where to die is often a problem facing patients and may raise many fears and concerns; this needs to be addressed sensitively and the patient allowed the time to express anxieties. The community palliative care clinical nurse specialist can make good use of her communication and interpersonal skills to assist the patient in decision making and to explore complex issues that the patient feels the need to address.

Case Story: Ian

Ian was in the last few weeks of his life. He had been asked on several occasions about place of death, but had never committed himself to home or hospice care. One day, when the community palliative care clinical nurse specialist visited and his wife was out shopping, Ian became very emotional and reported that his wish was to die at home. However, his wife had commented many years before when a neighbour died at home that the man should have been nursed in a hospice. She had reported that his wife was exhausted trying to care for her husband. He had always remembered this and did not know how to approach this topic with his own wife. He agreed for the community palliative care clinical nurse specialist to act as a facilitator in communicating with his wife regarding this emotional and sensitive subject. At a subsequent visit, Ian's wife agreed that she

---

had made those remarks previously, but reported that it was easy to make comments as a neighbour; her greatest wish now was that Ian should stay at home and allow her to care for him and that he should die at home.

It is sometimes difficult for individuals to express their problems, and establishing a relationship of trust with patients is essential to good palliative care. It also has to be remembered that patients will only reveal and discuss their problems if given the opportunity and encouragement to do so. As a consequence, health professionals who fail to ask appropriate questions or appear harassed and preoccupied may never get the *real* picture from their patients.

Case Story: Catherine

Catherine had lived with cancer for many years and knew that she was now in her last weeks of life. The general practitioner remarked to the community palliative care clinical nurse specialist that Catherine never complained about her situation or reported problematic symptoms; as a result the general practitioner visited rarely. The community palliative care clinical nurse specialist had visited Catherine regularly and found they were always lengthy visits. At these visits Catherine would express the pain of leaving her family and the injustice of life. She used to comment that it was good to have the opportunity to talk with the community palliative care clinical nurse specialist as other health professionals, especially the general practitioner, always seemed so busy and only asked about her pain; she did not like to bother them with her worries.

One of the most important aspects of caring for those with palliative care needs is to listen; this will establish the needs of the patient and subsequently allow the individual to retain as much control of the situation as possible, providing not only physical care, but also emotional support (Wells 2001).

People differ in how they respond to the prospect of death; however, fear of death and the process of dying are common and discussion about the management and care can often lead to a more realistic view of it. Most patients are understandably afraid of the unknown, such as dying in pain or losing control of bladder or bowels. As a result of our changing society, most individuals have little personal experience of death and it still remains a taboo subject for many people; therefore information and good communication are necessary to allay fears and allow patients to make choices in their care. The community palliative care clinical nurse specialist can assist patients in expressing their fears and give information as required. The psychological support and physical care required at this time can be considerable and, along with the primary health care team, the community palliative care clinical nurse specialist can assess the needs of these patients to provide optimum palliative care.

Key Points

- The diagnosis of a life-threatening illness can be devastating, with many patients unable to absorb the information being given.
- The community palliative care clinical nurse specialist is available to give information and also emotional and practical support to these patients, from the time of their diagnosis.
- Actively listening to patients may do much to allay their fears and allow them to express their emotions; the community palliative care clinical nurse specialist has the expertise and skills to provide the specialist care needed at this time.
- The role of the community palliative care clinical nurse specialist is to assist patients to understand what has been discussed with their doctors in regard to the treatment on offer, its potential benefits in relation to their disease, length of treatment and side-effects.
- After treatment, whether it is radiotherapy, chemotherapy or surgery, etc., the patient will require ongoing support for weeks, months or in some cases years.
- Many patients report that the news of recurrence is more difficult to cope with than the original diagnosis.
- The role of the community palliative care clinical specialist is multifaceted and flexibility is required to not only deal with support and information giving, but also facilitate patients in their emotional journey from curative treatments to palliative care.
- The support of these patients requires teamwork; the resources of the primary health care team and the community palliative care clinical nurse specialist working collaboratively, to ease the patient's journey.

Useful resources

Brennan J (2004) *Cancer in Context: A Practical Guide to Supportive Care.* Oxford University Press, Oxford.

Corner J, Bailey C (eds) (2001) *Cancer Nursing: Care in Context.* Blackwell Science, Oxford.

Lee E (2002) *In Your Own Time: A Guide for Patients and Their Carers Facing a Last Illness at Home.* Oxford University Press, Oxford.

Palmer E, Howarth J (2005) *Palliative Care for the Primary Care Team.* Quay Books, London.

Payne S, Seymour J, Ingleton C (eds) (2004) *Palliative Care Nursing: Principles and Evidence for Practice.* Open University Press, Maidenhead.

References

Akkerman D (1998) The importance of communication and the provision of information in patient care. In: Poulton G (ed) *Nursing the Person with Cancer: A Book for All Nurses*, pp 27–37. Ausmed, Ascot Vale Victoria.

Barraclough J (1999) *Cancer and Emotion: A Practical Guide to Psycho-Oncology*, 3rd edn. John Wiley and Sons, Chichester.

Blows WT (2005) *The Biological Basis of Nursing: Cancer.* Routledge, Abingdon.

Brennan J (2004) *Cancer in Context: A Practical Guide to Supportive Care.* Oxford University Press, Oxford.

Buckman R (1995) *What You Really Need to Know About Cancer.* Key Porter Books, Ontario.

Carr AJ, Gibson B, Robinson PG (2001) Is quality of life determined by expectations or experience? *British Medical Journal* 322, 1240–1243.

Cooper GM (1993) *The Cancer Book.* Jones and Bartlett, Boston.

Corner J, Kelly D (2001) The experience of treatment. In: Corner J, Bailey C (eds) *Cancer Nursing: Care in Context*, pp 143–155. Blackwell Science, Oxford.

Coyler H (2003) The context of radiotherapy care. In: Faithfull S, Wells M (eds) *Supportive Care in Radiotherapy*, pp 1–16. Churchill Livingstone, Edinburgh.

Davy J, Ellis S (2000) *Counselling Skills in Palliative Care.* Open University Press, Buckingham.

Doyle D, Jeffrey J (2000) *Palliative Care in the Home.* Oxford University Press, Oxford.

Faithfull S (2001) Radiotherapy. In: Corner J, Bailey C (2001) *Cancer Nursing: Care in Context*, pp 222–261. Blackwell Science, Oxford.

Faulkner A, Maguire P (1994) *Talking to Cancer Patients and Their Families.* Oxford University Press, Oxford.

Faull C, Barton R (1998) Managing complications of cancer. In: Faull C, Carter Y, Woof R (eds) *Handbook of Palliative Care,* pp 177–201. Blackwell Science, Oxford.

Faithful S (2001) Radiotherapy. In: Corner J, Bailey CD (eds) *Cancer Nursing: Care in Context,* pp 222–261. Blackwell Science, Oxford.

Groenwald SL, Frogge MH, Goodman M, Yarbro CH (1997) *Clinical Guide to Cancer Nursing,* 4th edn. Jones and Bartlett, Sudbury.

Hoskin P, Makin W (2003) *Oncology for Palliative Medicine,* 2nd edn. Oxford University Press, Oxford.

Jeffrey D (1998) Communication skills in palliative care. In: Faull C, Carter Y, Woof R (eds) (1998) *Handbook of Palliative Care,* pp 88–98. Blackwell Science, Oxford.

Jeffrey D (2000) *Cancer from Cure to Care: Palliative Care Dilemmas in General Practice.* Hochland and Hochland, Manchester.

Johnson BL, Gross J (1998) *Handbook of Oncology Nursing,* 3rd edn. Jones and Bartlett, Sudbury.

Lee E (2002) *In Your Own Time: A Guide for Patients and Their Carers Facing a Last Illness at Home.* Oxford University Press, Oxford.

Lloyd-Williams M (2004) Emotions and cognitions: Psychological aspects of care. In: Payne S, Seymour J, Ingleton C (eds) *Palliative Care Nursing: Principles and Evidence for Practice,* pp 299–311. Open University Press, Maidenhead.

Napier M, Srinivasan R (2002) Disease modifying treatments in palliative care. In: Penson J, Fisher RA (eds) (2002) *Palliative Care for People with Cancer,* 3rd edn, pp 154–167. Arnold, London.

Palmer E, Howarth J (2005) *Palliative Care for the Primary Care Team.* Quay Books, London.

Skilbeck J, Payne S (2004) Emotional support and the role of clinical nurse specialists in palliative care. *Journal of Advanced Nursing* 43 (5), 521–530.

Twycross R (1997) *Introducing Palliative Care,* 3rd edn. Radcliffe Medical Press, Abingdon.

Wells M (2001) The impact of cancer. In: Corner J, Bailey C (eds) *Cancer Nursing: Care in Context,* pp 63–85. Blackwell Science, Oxford.

Woof R, Carter Y, Harrison B, Faull C, Nyatanga B (1998) Terminal care and dying. In: Faull C, Carter Y, Woof R (eds) *Handbook of Palliative Care,* pp 307–332. Blackwell Science, Oxford.

Young W (2001) Breaking bad news. In: Gabriel J (ed) *Oncology Nursing in Practice,* pp 327–332. Whurr, London.

Life at Home

4

Introduction

The original concept of a National Health Service gradually producing a population of healthier individuals has never been realised (Hasler 1990). With the increasing efficiency of our health care system many lives have been saved, but this has also resulted in an ever-increasing number of chronic health problems (Altschuler et al. 1997; Curtin and Lubkin 1998). As a result of medical advances and the treatments available, many of the individuals faced with a life-threatening illness, such as cancer, can now be said to be suffering from a chronic illness.

What is the definition of a chronic illness? Chronic means *lingering* (Oxford Dictionary 1986) and an *illness* is the human experience of symptoms and suffering (Curtin and Lubkin 1998). According to Stoll (1998), a chronic illness is a long, unpredictable journey unique to the individual and affects relationships, roles and lifestyle. Patients with a chronic illness have to live their lives dealing with the personal, family and illness-related problems that each day brings. This has a major impact on not only the individuals, but also their families and the health services.

The Department of Health (2001) states that it wants to empower people living with a chronic illness to become decision makers in their own care, to work in partnership with health professionals and improve their overall quality of life. In today's political environment, the emphasis is firmly placed on the community and caring for patients within their own homes.

Family and social issues

Being unwell can be a disabling experience, both physically and psychologically, and may be accompanied by feelings of helplessness and loss of control (Hurdman 1995). Add to this situation the knowledge that the illness is life limiting and suddenly the patient's world that was familiar and secure becomes unpredictable and frightening. This impacts not only on the patient, but also on those around him or her and, in particular, the individuals the patient refers to as *family*.

In today's society, the meaning of family may be difficult to define and may be different to each person, depending on his/her personal situation and cultural background. The *family* may consist of partners, parents, siblings, children and close friends (Plant 2001). It may involve members from different generations or simply a lone parent with one child. What is important is the role the patient plays in the family and the impact of his or her illness on the normal functioning of that family. In the early stages of the illness there may be little impact on daily activities; however, the patient and family are now living with the uncertainty that the illness brings and also the knowledge of future separation. The patient and family will have many concerns: fear of the unknown, fear of pain and other symptoms, fear of the dying process, concerns about ability to cope, as well as feelings of depression, sadness and loneliness (Wilkie 1998).

Impact of illness on family life

The scope of technology today has extended the life of many patients; however, it also means that the disease trajectory is punctuated by periods of ill health and a slow gradual deterioration for many individuals. This will increase the patient's dependence not only on the health and social care services, but also on the members of the family. As a result, the patient and family may have to undergo many changes, some suddenly, some over a period of weeks or months, in response to the illness. The diagnosis of a life-threatening illness in one member of the family will subsequently and sadly affect all members of that family. The impact of the illness will depend on the role of the patient within the family prior to the illness; for example, the breadwinner in the family, the mother of young children, the carer of an elderly parent or an elderly spouse. The age of the patient will also have an impact on the family dynamics, for example the younger patient may be able to self care and be more independent, whilst the elderly may be coping with not only their life-threatening illness, but also other long-term conditions.

During the past century, life expectancy has increased markedly in the United Kingdom. This has resulted in a large rise in the elderly population, many of whom live healthier and more independent lives than previous generations (Barnett 2002). However, these demographic changes have also seen an increase in long-term health conditions, increasing expenditure on health care and the increased need for social and health services. As a result of the demographic changes, long-term care in the community for those with an ongoing illness is now required on a scale not previously imagined (Coote 1996). A diagnosis of cancer or other life-threatening illness can result in its own problems for the elderly age group, many of whom live alone. The increasing mobility of extended families and changes in working patterns, particularly for women, has meant that many elderly can no longer rely on family members to provide care and are now dependent on social, health and voluntary services to remain in their own homes. This can have a major impact on the primary health care team and the delivery of palliative care, particularly for those patients who express a desire to remain at home during their illness.

Case Story: Annabelle

Annabelle, a widow, had lived alone for 4 years. She had a very caring family, but unfortunately they all lived overseas and were unable to return home to be with Annabelle. Her cancer had been diagnosed not long after her husband's death, but she coped with the illness and maintained her independence. The house was remote, with no immediate neighbours and no transport link, making it more difficult for her elderly friends to visit. The community palliative care clinical nurse specialist had supported Annabelle for some time and had discussed on many occasions the challenge of providing daily care for Annabelle when her condition deteriorated. Annabelle was anxious about the loss of her independence and ability to stay at home. However, she fully understood the possible difficulties and was willing to accept help from health and social agencies. Through time, Annabelle became increasingly frail and the community palliative care clinical nurse specialist worked closely with the district nurse caring for Annabelle, coordinating visits and organising Marie Curie nurses, to allow Annabelle the security of nursing visits every day. Referral to the social services also provided assistance with personal

---

Case Story: Annabelle (*continued*)

hygiene, meal preparation, etc. Annabelle's care involved considerable input from all the services and at times this proved difficult to maintain; however, Annabelle felt secure and was happy to be able to remain in her own home.

Research by McKenzie et al. (2007) identified that patients feel less anxious and are more confident in their day-to-day lives when contact with the community nurses is regular and consistent. The coordinated visits by the community nursing staff to Annabelle certainly gave her confidence to remain at home and, although difficult at times, demonstrated the value of the nursing and social services working collaboratively as a team, to achieve the desired goal. The health and social services are the two agencies with the most responsibility for assisting patients at home; however, the line between social and health care can be hard to draw exactly and difficulties can emerge (Coote 1996). The changes within the district nursing services in recent years have seen, in the absence of other nursing needs, help with personal hygiene as no longer part of the nursing role. This once core facet of nursing work has been relabelled as social care provision. This can create difficulties for some elderly patients who have traditionally thought of the nurse as providing personal care and at times resent the intrusion of the *social services*. Careful explanation is required to facilitate understanding of the differing roles within the community and ensure patients are in receipt of the services most appropriate to their needs, to allow them to remain within their own homes during their illness.

However, for some older patients the wish to remain at home during their illness is not always possible.

Case Story: Joseph

Joseph had lung cancer. He lived alone, but had two daughters who lived locally. His condition changed when he was diagnosed with cerebral metastases. Initially the support from social services and input from his daughters was sufficient to maintain Joseph at home. However, he started to have falls and his daughters were struggling to cope. The community palliative care clinical nurse specialist was asked to visit to offer support to Joseph and his daughters. She discovered that the daughters were also caring for their mother (divorced from Joseph many years before) and that their mother had dementia. Both daughters were upset at the impending loss of their father and their inability to care for him. They both felt physically and emotionally drained. Despite full services from health and social care, Joseph was still at risk and he also reported feeling a burden to his daughters. Joseph was already thinking about a nursing home, but was unsure how to raise the subject with his daughters. His wish had always been to remain at home and both his daughters had promised their father that they would care for him. The community palliative care clinical nurse specialist facilitated a meeting with all the relevant parties. Joseph felt relieved when his daughters agreed to him moving to a local nursing home.

The role of the community palliative care clinical nurse specialist is to act as facilitator when families find communication difficult. At times, it is merely allowing everyone to express their feelings and bring situations 'out into the open'. Patients are often concerned about the extra demands their illness makes on family members, none more so than when the spouse is also an older person. Many elderly are quite isolated as families do not live nearby and their friends are also of a similar age to themselves and less able to offer help (Wilkie 1998). The incidence of cancer rises with age, as does other conditions such as arthritis, hypertension, diabetes, angina, and visual and hearing impairments (Brennan 2004); therefore, the older person may be less able to carry out activities around the home and self care, even before the diagnosis of a life-threatening condition. Assessment from the community palliative care clinical nurse specialist has to take into account all of these factors and therefore explores not only the complex psychological issues which the patient may identify, but also the more practical problems. This requires collaboration with other members of the primary health care team and other agencies to meet the needs of the patient.

Adapting to change

Younger patients with a life-threatening illness will face their own challenges whilst living at home. Successful adaptation to any illness includes developing coping strategies to deal with the stressors produced by the uncertainty and demands of the illness. White et al. (1992) found that coping efforts may be directed outward toward changing the environment (problem focused) or inward toward changing the meaning of the event (emotion focused). A problem-focused approach will see the patient clarifying the problem, identifying changes to accommodate the problem, looking at all the options and taking action. An emotion-focused approach results in avoidance, distancing themselves from the issue, venting feelings of anger, aggression or indeed violence.

The community palliative care clinical nurse specialist has an understanding of the adaptation process and can assist the patient to plan effective interventions which will enable psychosocial adaptation (Whyte 1997). Patients' reactions to illness will also depend on other factors, for example their own personal experience of the disease and people they have known or heard about with the same illness (Bendall and Muncey 2002), the level of perceived support available to them, i.e. the greater the support, the better the psychosocial adjustment to the illness (White et al. 1992), and the characteristics of the disease, degree of disability and extent of medical intervention required (Curtin and Lubkin 1998). Often the prognosis in a life-threatening illness is unclear and only as the disease progresses is it possible to estimate what will transpire. This can be particularly difficult for younger patients who have major life decisions ahead of them (Strauss et al. 1984). With a life-threatening illness the patient can be left feeling powerless. This can result in apathy, withdrawal, isolation and a lack of motivation (Deegan 1996). In order to balance a sense of hope with acceptance, people need to be empowered to make choices about their ongoing care and be helped with coping strategies to accept their illness and its uncertainty.

People who live with an ongoing disease do most of the work associated with managing the illness themselves (Crumbie 2002). Being at home allows patients to have greater autonomy and more control over their care. The main focus for those with a life-threatening illness is not just to stay alive or keep their symptoms under control, but to live as normally as possible. This will include encountering many of the daily problems such as loss of productive functioning, financial strain, employment issues, family stress, personal distress (spirituality), stigma, changes in physical appearance, a restricted life leading to isolation, fears and anxieties about pain, and countless hospital and related appointments.

Living with loss

All patients with a life-threatening condition face losses and these are often associated with their life at home. The losses experienced by patients often begin from the time of diagnosis. Many patients will have had to give up work, with the ensuing financial consequences due to not only loss of income, but also the added extra expense of heating the home during their illness, travel costs to the hospital, prescription charges, etc. Patients may also experience a role change within the home, loss of social contacts and loss of social position. Not only do they have to cope with the loss of their physical health and the difficulties it brings, but also they may experience loss of their family role.

Case Story: Derek

Derek worked on a farm and had always been the main wage earner in the family. He had two young sons and his wife worked only a few hours each week. He was diagnosed with a brain tumour and had to give up work and driving. His wife managed to increase her hours of work to help their finances. After his surgery, Derek was initially well and looked after their sons. Through time his condition deteriorated and gradually he was less able to care for himself. His dependence on his wife increased and she had to give up her work to care for him. He realised that his two young sons were distancing themselves from their father, partly because of their fear of his frequent seizures, but they were also being asked to do more around the home, as their mother struggled to cope. Derek also reported a loss of 'closeness' with his wife. He became very depressed and reported feeling useless. He no longer saw his role as that of a father or a husband.

Feelings of uselessness can arise from the physical, emotional or social limitations that come with a life-threatening illness (Kemp 1999). Identification of the patient's complex emotional state by the general practitioner or other member of the primary health care team normally initiates referral to the community palliative care clinical nurse specialist. The specialist's role is to assist the patient to overcome these complex feelings and emotions, through strategies adapted for the patient. By asking the family to involve the patient in decision making, the patient can feel again that his or her opinion is valued, by being more involved in family activities, however limited; once again, this creates a feeling of belonging to the family, and by encouraging the family and patient to share their feelings, in particular their feelings of loss, this may achieve resolution or acceptance (Kemp 1999).

Body image and sexuality

Living with an ongoing illness may present other problems at home. The patient's loss of independence can lead to a confined lifestyle where the individual becomes effectively housebound (Radley 1994). This can have a potentially devastating outcome for any individual, regardless of age. Loss of social integration can lead to loneliness and depression, resulting in low energy, fatigue and decreased libido (Larsen et al. 1998). Sexuality and sexual relationships are basic to social life and a life-threatening illness may alter one's perceptions of self as a sexual being.

For many health professionals, consideration of sexuality in a palliative care setting can feel inappropriate or awkward (Palmer and Howarth 2005). However, at home, this may give rise to many problems and, as the above patient described, a lack of *closeness* to his wife. Issues of intimacy and sexuality are about considerably more than acts of intercourse (Monroe and Sheldon 2004). Sexuality can mean companionship, love, intimacy or sexual activity and can be affected by illness through lack of sexual function, body image changes or decreased libido. Many of these problems will be as a result of the cancer treatments or surgery; for example, patients may be dealing with hair loss, stoma formation, mastectomy scarring, pelvic surgery or treatment to head and neck tumours causing disfigurement. Partners may find that physical changes in the patient have altered their own feelings and sexual desires (Monroe and Sheldon 2004). This may further isolate the patient from the love and support needed at this time. Add to this the physical symptoms of fatigue, pain, nausea, constipation and breathlessness, etc. and it becomes apparent why patients may have difficulty with sexuality.

For some patients, the diagnosis of cancer and its treatments can have a marked negative effect on body image and subsequent sexuality. Changes in body image can and do become psychological barriers in sexual relationships (Kelly 1992). Body image relates partly to the appearance of the body, but also to how the patient visualises his or her own body (Palmer and Howarth 2005). Effects of the cancer may result in muscle wasting, cachexia or jaundice, with the patient very self-conscious of the changes. Adjusting to changes in body image can prove difficult and also requires those close to the patient to attempt to adjust to the new image. Addressing the impact of body image change is as important as acknowledging symptoms (Dryden 2003) and health care professionals, such as the community palliative care clinical nurse specialist, can make a difference to body image problems through careful assessment and sensitive management.

Case Story: Marilyn

Marilyn was 43 years of age and had always been proud of her hour-glass figure, her long hair and pretty face. This had changed in the last few months after she was diagnosed with breast cancer. She had had a right mastectomy, followed by chemotherapy. She could not bring herself to allow her husband into the same bed and their marital relationship was deteriorating. She would not talk to her husband about the situation. He asked the general practitioner for help. The community palliative care clinical nurse specialist was asked to visit the couple. The role of the community palliative care clinical nurse specialist was to act as facilitator and encourage the couple to start communicating about their feelings. Marilyn was initially reluctant to discuss the problems with her husband. However, gradually her husband helped her to express how she felt. Marilyn expressed her disgust at the way she looked. She felt mutilated, had no hair, no energy and no longer felt that she was a wife. After several very emotional and distraught visits the couple were discussing their emotions openly. Marilyn was helped to realise that her husband continued to love her and he himself admitted he had had to adapt to her new image. Their marital relationship improved and eventually they both felt they had rekindled the feelings that had been missing for several months.

Learning to ask about sexual health is part of the health care professionals' responsibilities (Burton and Watson 1998) and part of the role of the community palliative care clinical nurse specialist. The nurse's purpose is not to provide sex therapy, but rather to identify problems and try to support the patient in coping with the problems (Kemp 1999). Anxiety and fear, particularly about dying, can alter patients' attitudes to their sexuality and the need for intimacy. However, as an illness progresses the patient may feel an increased need for physical touch, and the partner should be encouraged to hold a hand, to cuddle or simply to lie beside his or her loved one. The comfort given by simple touch can help to alleviate the loss of intimacy experienced by patients at this time. Intimacy and privacy are easier to maintain at home and therefore expressions of sexuality or sexual relationships may be easier preserved within familiar surroundings (Arras and Dubler 1995).

The community palliative care clinical nurse specialist can offer support and understanding to the patients and, by exploring this sensitive topic, will allow patients to express their emotions and bring the problem into the open. It is communication between patients and partners that is required to re-establish their intimacy, and the community palliative care clinical nurse specialist can act as facilitator in the communication process to address these complex needs.

Family communications

Communication plays an important part in caring for patients with a life-threatening illness. This involves dialogue both with patients and between patients and their families. In complex situations, where communication difficulties may have arisen, referral to the community palliative care clinical nurse specialist can be appropriate to discuss problems and facilitate the communication process between patients and their spouses or families. At times, patients try to shield family members from the truth about their illness; they dread having to answer difficult questions or having to cope with the tears and emotions (Doyle and Jeffrey 2000). In order to protect one another from hurt, it may seem safer to avoid talking about their emotions and difficult issues (Monroe and Sheldon 2004) and try to struggle on as if nothing is different in their lives. However, not speaking about what is happening cannot make the reality of the situation disappear. Talking about a life-threatening illness, its implications and the difficulties associated with it is difficult; even the closest of relationships may have difficulty in sharing their concerns, fears and anxieties (Plant 2001). This may lead to feelings of loneliness and isolation. Patients and their families need encouragement to discuss issues openly and sensitively; this will be preferable to the feelings of isolation, uncertainty and suspicion of not communicating about the illness and the future.

Communicating with children

Communication is important between patients, their partners, their families and their children. However, many find talking with their children, about their illness and impending death, particularly difficult. Many patients and their families try to exclude children and grandchildren from involvement with the patient and his/her illness, hoping to protect them from distress (Oliver 2000). However, children will realise that something is wrong and need to be given information appropriate to their age and maturity. Lee (2002) reports that children are aware that something is wrong whether or not they are told; they see a parent upset or ill and this can make them feel lonely and afraid.

Given the enormity of the information they may have to impart, many parents worry about the effect it will have on their children (Brennan 2004). The community palliative care clinical nurse specialist can reassure patients that they will instinctively know what to tell their children, to be as honest and open as possible and give the children time to absorb the information and allow a further opportunity to ask questions. If children are not told what is happening to their father or mother, they may create their own ideas and become worried or anxious that they are somehow to blame for what is happening. Above all, children need to know that they are loved, that they will be looked after and not abandoned. These issues can be especially difficult for single parents who may have to arrange the future care of their child or children.

Case Story: Amy

Amy (26) was diagnosed with gastric cancer when her daughter Laura was 4 years old. Laura's father had not been around since his daughter's birth and his whereabouts were not known. Amy had to deal with the turmoil of her surgery, chemotherapy and uncertain future, whilst caring for her daughter. She asked for assistance from the community palliative care clinical nurse specialist in communicating with her daughter. As well as offering support, the community palliative care clinical nurse specialist gave Amy written information on communicating with children. This she was able to read and absorb in her own time. Amy decided that she would only discuss the cancer with Laura and not discuss death at this stage. Instinctively she felt that Laura would not fully understand the concept of death at this time and Amy was still hoping for a successful outcome from her treatments. She reported that if her condition changed, she would then talk to Laura about death. Amy reported that speaking to Laura had been easier than she had imagined and that the little girl had

Case Story: Amy (*continued*)

asked very sensible questions. Her main concern was to gain reassurance that her grandmother would know how to care for her should the need arise.

The instincts of parents are to protect their children, and when someone is very ill or dying, the urge is to shield children from the situation (Kemp 1998); however, children should be told the truth about illness and death. The amount of information given will be dependent on the age of the children and their ability to comprehend what is being relayed to them. Parents often need help to break bad news to their children. The community palliative care clinical nurse specialist can support parents and offer advice on communicating with children, and in some circumstances can facilitate a meeting with parents and their children to discuss complex issues and answer questions. Referral on to a social worker, with particular interest in child care, may be invaluable in helping both the parents and the children to talk about the illness and the future (Oliver 2000). Patients will also want to continue to care for their children and it is important to support them in this endeavour for as long as possible, ensuring that referral on to other agencies is discussed and back-up is organised for when the parent becomes unwell.

Quality of life

Life at home can become very difficult for patients when they are unwell, for a variety of reasons. Many patients will show the community palliative care clinical nurse specialist their diary and, sadly, most of the contacts over the months are with health care professionals, either at the hospital or visiting the house. This places a strain on the household because of the need to plan each day and each journey, particularly if the hospital is some distance from home. It removes the spontaneity of seeing the sun shining and deciding to go out for lunch or to have friends to the house for a meal. Patients often report to the community palliative care clinical nurse specialist that the illness takes over their life. It therefore takes its toll not only on the patient, but also on the family. They are unable to plan ahead, unsure how the patient will feel on a particular day, unable to say *yes* to friends' invitations or plan any holidays in advance. Patients and their families need to be given the opportunity to discuss these issues and express the complex emotions they are experiencing. The community palliative care clinical nurse specialist can assist the patient and family to review their hospital visits, negotiate with departments over their clinic appointment times to fit more easily with the family schedule, and coordinate visits to the home from other health care professionals. These simple measures may make a considerable difference to the quality of life of patients and allow them to regain some control over their day-to-day activities.

Case Story: Hilary

Hilary enjoyed playing golf, but over the past few months this had been more difficult due to Christopher's illness. Her husband had considerable fatigue and found his energy was needed for visits to the doctor's surgery, hospital and local clinic for physiotherapy. He was also being visited at home by the community nurses and occupational therapist. He found it all overwhelming and asked his wife to be at home for their visits. Christopher expressed feelings of guilt because his wife was staying at home and missing out on her normal social activities. At times he felt a burden to his wife. The community palliative care clinical nurse specialist listened to Christopher's concerns and allowed him to express his emotions. After discussion with his wife, it was decided to negotiate the contacts with the other health professionals involved in his care to try to streamline his home visits and trips to hospital, etc. to one or two days per week. He agreed to attend the local specialist palliative day care facility, where he would be able to meet with the physiotherapist and attend a fatigue workshop; this would also allow his wife one planned day per week when she could golf with her friends. Christopher found his fatigue improved due to a more relaxed weekly schedule and he enjoyed his weekly visit to the day care unit.

Quality of life is a vague concept and what constitutes quality of life ultimately remains philosophical (Bowling 1995). Problems are encountered when trying to measure health-related quality of life, as patients have different expectations and responses to illness (Carr et al. 2001). The role of the community palliative care clinical nurse specialist is to assist patients to adjust their expectations and facilitate adaptation to their changed status.

Adapting to loss

When patients are diagnosed with cancer or other life-threatening ill-ness there will be inevitable changes in their daily routines. Younger patients have to cope with the loss of employment due to their inabil-ity to work. This also brings about the loss of contact with work col-leagues and, at times, the loss of friends, the loss of their career and social status, accompanied by the loss of future plans. Individuals may also experience a lack of structure to their day and resulting feelings of boredom and frustration. Information and support are needed to restore their sense of dignity and self worth through decision making and regaining control wherever possible (Monroe and Sheldon 2004). The community palliative care clinical nurse specialist can encourage patients to express their feelings of loss and offer support and strategies for maintaining contact with friends and colleagues; perhaps through the simple use of e-mail or by telephone. Unfortunately, as an illness progresses patients usually have to give up driving and, consequently, the loss of their independence in mobility, thus increasing their sense of social isolation.

Case Story: Hugh

Hugh worked in a physically demanding job prior to his diagnosis of lung cancer. He had always been 'one of the lads' and enjoyed a busy social life with his work colleagues. He had lost several stones in weight at the start of his illness and found difficulties with his subsequent body image. He reported that 'the lads' did not ask him out any more and did not visit the house. He felt very alone and angry at his friends for abandoning him. The community palliative care clinical nurse specialist allowed Hugh to express his feelings and acknowledged his anger. It was apparent after talking to Hugh that some of his friends had indeed been contacting the house and invit-ing him to join them, but Hugh had declined their invitations. He reported feeling detached from his friends, his physical appearance was also different and he was yearning for his previous life.

Not everyone experiences all of these losses, but most patients will have to cope with some loss. A life-threatening illness, such as can-cer, involves a whole series of losses; health care professionals need to be aware of the different kinds of loss that patients may experience

(Davy and Ellis 2000). As well as the loss of their physical health, they may experience the loss of emotional well-being, loss of independence and loss of self care (Palmer and Howarth 2005). With a life-threatening illness, the patient has limited time to adapt to one loss when another may surface. The natural response to loss is grief. The power of grief should not be underestimated by health care professionals, as it has a profound effect on patients and their families (Kemp 1999).

The reactions to grief are similar to the reactions of being given bad news. There may be the initial shock and numbness, followed by anger, guilt, anxiety and sadness. The feelings and emotions associated with loss and grief are not static but complex and patients may shift between the different emotions in short periods of time (Palmer and Howarth 2005). The role of the community palliative care clinical nurse specialist is to assist patients in recognising and adapting to their loss and grief. The first step is to acknowledge the loss and its significance to the patient, thus demonstrating an understanding of what he or she is experiencing. It may also be necessary to help the patient explore the loss and its meaning and, where necessary, to facilitate the patient to adjust to the loss.

Spirituality

Patients with a life-threatening illness face not only loss, but also suffering, helplessness, fear and at times despair. Although these feelings may arise from the physical illness and its related symptoms, the patient may also be experiencing spiritual distress. In order to increase the quality of life of a patient with a life-threatening illness, all aspects of the patient (mind, body and spirit) should be addressed (Hermann 2001). The importance of spirituality is recognised within palliative care and helping patients to address the spiritual aspects of their lives offers the health care professional an opportunity to deliver truly holistic care.

Spirituality is concerned with how individuals understand the purpose and meaning of their existence within this world (Woof and Nyatanga 1998) and examines what we are, rather than what we do. Carson (1998) describes spirituality as a dynamic process in which the person becomes aware of the meaning, purpose and values in his or her life. In order to alleviate spiritual distress, the community palliative care clinical nurse specialist may have to offer assistance and support to allow patients to address unresolved difficult family relationships or simply to listen to the questions that are troubling them. The patient may have many questions, most of which have no clear answers. For example: Why me? What have I done to deserve this? Why now? Although no answers may be possible, it is important to listen to patients and acknowledge their questions and how they are feeling.

Case Story: Craig

Craig was a young man with a brain tumour. He had surgery and radiotherapy, but his treatment was of palliative intent and Craig was aware that he would die one day from the tumour. He had lived a very full life and admitted to enjoying a few beers, smoking a bit of dope and liking the company of good-looking women. But now his mobility was poor, he was always tired and he experienced occasional seizures. He no longer joined his friends to socialise and became very quiet and withdrawn. One day, whilst talking to the community palliative care clinical nurse specialist, he broke down and sobbed. He felt angry with life: why had this happened to him and who could explain it? He could not understand it and cried, 'I have never done anyone any harm. I've never been in trouble. I've always been a good lad'.

The community palliative care clinical nurse specialist is ideally placed to help the patient who is spiritually distressed, having the skills and competency in dealing with spiritual care. Unfortunately, other members of the health care team may not have had the learning opportunities that are available to the community palliative care clinical nurse specialist and therefore may struggle with this aspect of palliative care. A study by Ross (1994) found that the spiritual needs of some patients may go unrecognised or may be dealt with inappropriately. One of the problems in addressing spiritual care with patients is that many of the health professionals making the assessment are unclear about their own spiritual beliefs (Speck 2004). This calls for the effectiveness of teamwork within primary care in recognising that another member of the team may have the skills required to deal with particular complex issues. The community palliative care clinical nurse specialist can provide spiritual care by listening to patients, acknowledging their distress and offering them support and reassurance.

Many everyday things can do much to 'lift the spirit' and enrich lives; a gift of flowers, a letter from a friend, a smile, or love and support from someone close (Booth 2000). Spiritual care can be provided by simply being with the patient; however, the spiritual needs of individuals facing a life-threatening illness may vary greatly and can also impact on other presenting problems (Hunt et al. 2003). Spiritual distress itself may present as constant worrying, anxiety, depression and insomnia. There will also be instances where the community palliative care clinical nurse specialist identifies that referral on to a psychologist may be necessary for more specialised care.

In some cultures there is a strong link between spirituality and religion. Spirituality may or may not have a religious component, but it is not necessary for the health care professional to hold similar beliefs or agree with the beliefs of the patient in order to meet the patient's spiritual needs with understanding and acceptance (Gerardi 1989). For many patients, religious belief has considerable significance as they journey towards the end of their life. It is not uncommon for spirituality to be expressed through religious activities such as prayers and church services. Patients who have religious beliefs are often greatly helped by the support offered by chaplains and priests. Some individuals may be experiencing fears that God has abandoned them or that their illness may be as a result of wrong-doings in their life. The availability of skilled help allows the patient to resolve difficulties and find peace of mind (Booth 2000).

In today's multicultural society it is important for health care professionals to be aware of the religious practices of patients and to respect the diversity of ethnic communities and their beliefs and rituals. It is important to recognise that when patients are facing a life-threatening illness, they experience a time of turmoil and powerful emotions (Clark 2002) and therefore it is essential to allow them to participate in their familiar practices and prayers to assist them with their spiritual needs. Patients living at home may feel more secure and have more privacy to express their spirituality and continue to fulfil religious obligations.

As demonstrated, life at home for the patient can be fraught with many difficulties; such as facing loss, changing roles, increasing dependence, issues with sexuality, communication difficulties and spiritual distress. This is by no means a comprehensive list of all the problems a patient may encounter, only some of the issues that may be raised. Add to this the investigations, treatments, hospital visits and domiciliary contacts from other health care professionals and it is easy to visualise a world where the patient feels he/she has lost control. Working alongside the other members of the primary health care team, the community palliative care clinical nurse specialist can support patients through their emotional journey and help them to regain some control over their lives. Unfortunately, patients will also have to address the many day-to-day practical problems that emerge as a result of their illness; the community palliative care clinical nurse specialist can also support the patient in managing the complex practical needs of living at home.

Practical problems

With improved survival rates, many life-threatening conditions are now becoming regarded as chronic illnesses (Brennan 2004). Even those patients who do not have a good prognosis are living longer and treatment is aimed at controlling the symptoms related to their disease (O'Neill and Leedham 2001). This presents many difficulties for patients who may have ongoing physical and emotional problems throughout their illness trajectory. The focus of supportive care for these patients is to restore quality of life and maximise physical function within the limits of their disease.

Case Story: Emily

Emily had breast cancer diagnosed at the age of 56. She was discovered to have bone metastases some years later after a pathological fracture of her right arm. This was slow to heal and resulted in some loss of function in her arm. After treatment, her cancer appeared to be stable. She was referred to the community palliative care clinical nurse specialist 8 years later when further bone deposits were discovered in her spine and pelvis, creating difficulties with mobility. Emily had lived with the illness, the uncertainty of her future and ongoing treatment for many years. However, what she found most difficult were the practical problems that arose as a result of the reduced function in her arm and then subsequently her mobility difficulties due to the spread of the disease. The role of the community palliative care clinical nurse specialist was to support Emily emotionally, but there was also a need to refer Emily on to the appropriate services to assist with her practical problems.

Offering support: emotional and practical

In order for the community palliative care clinical nurse specialist to access patients, a referral has to be generated from another health care professional, usually from the primary health care team. It is incumbent on the community palliative care clinical nurse specialist to ensure that other health care professionals are aware of the role and the specialist support that can be offered. The role of the community palliative care clinical nurse specialist in supporting the patient is complex and variable. Not only have patients to cope with the physical, psychological, spiritual and social effects of their illness, but also they have to adapt to the practical problems that ensue as a result of their changing needs. Increasing dependency is a difficult concept for many patients to conceive; they may have given thought to symptoms and the progression of their illness, but few will think about needing help to toilet, move in their own bed, personal hygiene or cleaning their own teeth. The demands imposed by the illness affect every aspect of the patient's life and can never be eliminated or forgotten (Turton and Orr 1993). The patient may have endured extended treatment over many months, followed by periods of recovery and then relapse. This is all accompanied by the psychological trauma of having a life-limiting illness and living at home with the debilitating effects of the disease.

Most written texts concentrate on the psychological effects of diagnosis and then again on the care of the patient who is dying, but for patients living with cancer or other life-threatening illness, the journey between diagnosis and death can be long and difficult. During this period of the illness, when their disease is more stable or when deterioration is very gradual, patients may have less contact with health care professionals, both within the secondary and primary care settings. However, the community palliative care clinical nurse specialist may continue to give emotional support to patients during this time and many patients may also need reassurance and support in making the practical changes that are necessary as their condition changes and impacts on their personal and social lives.

Subtle, gradual changes in a patient's condition may necessitate increased practical help. It is never possible to accurately predict how the illness will progress on a day-to-day or week-to-week basis and as a result the patient is constantly facing new challenges (McKenzie et al. 2007); at times these can seem overwhelming without support from health care professionals. When assessing the patient at home, the community palliative care clinical nurse specialist takes into account the normal daily routine of the individual and the household. Many of the practical problems encountered will require referral on to other disciplines and services: for example, district nurse, occupational therapist, physiotherapist, social worker. Communication with other members of the health care team is essential to ensure the patient receives all the help required as the illness progresses. Collaboration with colleagues can also raise standards of care by facilitating exchange of ideas, knowledge and previous experience (Woof et al.1998). Services should be requested promptly before a crisis arises, thereby allowing the patient to make the psychological adjustment to increased assistance as easy as possible.

Recognition is given to the fact that the physical and psychological problems associated with illness cannot be separated in a simple way and for most individuals the experience of illness is a complex association of physical, psychological and social issues (Payne and Ellis-Hill 2001).

Many patients regard interventions from other services and supply of equipment as a loss of independence; however, it is important that patients understand that supportive equipment and assistance from others allows them to remain at home and therefore increases their ability to live independently. Being at home allows patients greater choice in their supportive care and a semblance of control over the situation (Lee 2002). Many of the practical problems that patients encounter involve managing the routine activities of daily life such as dressing, bathing, toileting, cooking, laundry needs and shopping (Brennan 2004). These activities may have to be achieved when the patient is also suffering from physical symptoms such as fatigue and reduced energy levels, pain and discomfort or other debilitating problems.

Case Story: Judith

Judith was approaching her 90th birthday and lived alone. She had required no help around the house prior to her diagnosis of pancreatic cancer. Her main complaint was of overwhelming fatigue and she found even the slightest exertion exhausting. Having been independent, she was angry at the suggestion by the community palliative care clinical nurse specialist of help in the house. However, as her condition continued to deteriorate she reluctantly agreed to help with housework. This proved very successful and Judith soon agreed to assistance with meal preparation and shortly afterwards asked if she could have help with her personal hygiene. This allowed Judith to use her limited energy to enjoy the company of her friends.

The community palliative care clinical nurse specialist requires an extensive knowledge of the services and agencies available to patients in the community and frequently collaborates with the district nurse in the ongoing assessment of patients and their subsequent referral to other services. The assessment should centre on the patient's functional ability. For some patients, referral to the occupational therapist may be necessary for toileting and bathing aids. This may allow a patient to maintain independence in the bathroom, preserving privacy and dignity. Pieces of equipment such as a perching stool may allow an individual to participate in meal preparation in the kitchen and feel inclusive in family life. Referral to social services may be required to provide assistance with both personal care and meal preparation for patients unable to carry out these activities independently. Encouragement can be given to moving pieces of furniture, to allow easier and safer access to essential areas, such as the bed in the living room or a commode supplied to assist with toileting. For others, mobility may be challenging and again the occupational therapist may initiate the installation of ramps to allow access outdoors, whilst the physiotherapist can provide aids to assist with mobility.

The aim should be to restore function, promote independence and improve quality of life. The community palliative care clinical nurse specialist can provide support to the patient during this difficult time, when the individual may feel the loss of independence and increasing debility overwhelming. Allowing patients to express their feelings and gradually adapt to their changing condition may alleviate some of the stress and frustration within the home.

Safety is always a concern for vulnerable patients, especially for those living on their own. Referral to the social services for a community alarm may increase confidence in summoning assistance should the need arise, and features such as a key safe will allow carers to gain access safely and securely to a patient's home. Medication compliance may also be of concern to the community palliative care clinical nurse specialist, especially in the elderly; again social services can provide carers to assist with medication prompting. This essential service can ensure medication is taken as prescribed and help alleviate problematic, physical symptoms. Other patients will benefit from referral to the community pharmacist for a drug *dosette* box to be filled and dispensed weekly. This avoids confusion in the elderly, regarding the frequency and amounts of medication to be taken.

Case Story: George

George lived alone and reported that he did not like taking medication. He continually complained to his family about his symptoms,

> **Case Story:** George (*continued*)
>
> particularly pain and nausea. They in turn became angry with the health care professionals because of their perceived lack of action in controlling his persistent symptoms. The community palliative care clinical nurse specialist was asked to visit George and speak to his family. The family were unaware that George did not take his prescribed medication and asked for something to be done to resolve the situation. After discussion with other members of the primary health care team, it was agreed to refer George to the community pharmacist for a dosette box, to be delivered to the house weekly. This proved unsuccessful in persuading George to take his medication, but the family were then aware of the daily medications in the box being left untouched. His general condition had changed and it was agreed with George and his family to have carers in daily to assist with meal preparation; they were also asked to check if George had taken his medicines. With a little prompting, persuasion and perseverance George eventually started to take his prescribed analgesia and found that he became more mobile as his pain improved considerably.

Age-related problems

According to McMurray (2004), younger patients are often perceived to have more complex problems than the elderly; however, the elderly have problems that not only are related to their disease, but also may be specifically age related and associated with other chronic conditions. Difficulties that face elderly patients may also stem from the relationship they have with their respective spouse. For many, this will be the first time they have had to adapt their traditional role within the marriage. It may be difficult for an elderly husband to learn to cook and perhaps care for a house when his wife becomes unwell. And it can be equally difficult for an elderly wife to learn financial skills if her husband has always dealt with their money matters. The elderly require just as much support during their illness from the community palliative care clinical nurse specialist as younger patients; however. this support may be of a different nature, but the need is as great.

Younger patients may have very different practical problems at home, which need to be addressed: for example, someone to collect the children from school whilst the mother or father has treatment at the hospital; or to take care of the children during school holidays, if one parent is unwell. The community palliative care clinical nurse specialist needs to have the experience and knowledge to refer to the appropriate services, allowing patients to feel confident that their children are being cared for whilst they are unwell.

***

Case Story: Anita

Anita had 3-year-old twins and was receiving treatment for breast cancer. She had to plan her days around the nursery timetable, as she was adamant the girls should not have their normal routine disturbed. However, a change in treatment meant that she would not be home from hospital in time to collect them herself. With no family locally to help, Anita was torn between having the treatment and caring for her daughters. After discussion with the community palliative care clinical nurse specialist, Anita was referred to the social worker who organised for the girls to be collected from nursery and looked after until their mother arrived home. This was a great relief to Anita and allowed her to complete her treatment.

***

For some younger individuals, like Anita, the patient him-/herself may be a carer or have dependent family members. They may have children, elderly parents or elderly neighbours whom they have cared for over a period of time. Consideration needs to be given to relieving the burden of caring from these patients to allow them to concentrate on their own quality of life. The community palliative care clinical nurse specialist will take into account the role of the patient as a carer when undertaking the specialist nursing assessment and make referral to other agencies for assistance.

Financial concerns

Patients with a life-threatening illness have to cope with financial as well as medical problems as a result of their illness. Financial considerations, due to loss of income, weigh heavily on patients who have had to give up employment due to ill health. Younger patients may be anxious about the possibility of returning to work, unsure if they can still perform their job (Brennan 2004), and may face the prospect of unemployment with ensuing financial difficulties. Employment is not only a source of income, but also an essential component of normal life for many individuals (Cooper 1993). As stated previously, a life-threatening illness affecting one family member will impact on the others within the family. If the father/mother is unable to work then the whole family will be affected financially and also have to cope with him/her being at home all day (Turton and Orr 1993). Financial worries may contribute to the increasing burden that the illness is placing on the patient. There may be extra heating costs, prescription charges, the purchase of bedding and clothing (due to weight loss or weight gain), and for those patients below state pension age there will also be means-tested charges from the social services department for personal care, etc. given by their home carers.

The opportunity to discuss these issues and the chance to talk through their options may bring considerable relief to patients. For many, this will be their first encounter with the state welfare benefit system, which can be confusing and difficult to negotiate. Many state benefits are designed as short-term provision for the seriously ill, but many patients will have employment difficulties for months and even years (O'Neill and Leedham 2001). Referral by the community palliative care clinical nurse specialist to a medical social worker or local Welfare Rights department can assist the patient in making appropriate claims and completing the often incomprehensible forms. Completing a benefit claim form can be a painful experience and forces patients to face the reality, *in black and white*, of their diagnosis. This requires a supportive health care professional to acknowledge the patient's feelings and provide assistance in a sensitive manner. Other sources of financial support, which can be accessed by the community palliative care clinical nurse specialist, include charities (particularly Macmillan Cancer Support) which provide funds for heating and clothing, holidays or other needs which can be interpreted as improving the quality of life (Hurdman 1995).

Case Story: Michael

Michael had been unable to work for several years due to his cancer. He had two young daughters and his wife had a part-time job in a local shop. They had been surviving financially on state benefits and his wife's earnings. When his condition started to deteriorate his wife had to give up work to care for him. Their financial situation now deteriorated and his wife had to borrow money from a relative to pay heating fuel costs. Christmas was approaching and they were both distraught at being unable to provide presents for their daughters. Michael became depressed and a referral was made to the community palliative care clinical nurse specialist to offer the couple support. Michael confided to the nurse their financial problems and she contacted Welfare Rights to review their state benefits. Welfare Rights discovered Michael and his wife were not receiving their full entitlement of state benefits and would be entitled to more weekly income. A cancer charity was approached and the award of a financial grant also helped to ease their situation.

Financial difficulties undoubtedly contribute to an already distressing situation (Rose 2001), with the loss of income markedly affecting quality of life for patients and their families. The role of the community palliative care clinical nurse specialist is to empower the patient by providing information regarding state benefits and to ensure referral is made to the appropriate agencies to provide assistance.

Social isolation and the family

Other problems that may also cause practical difficulties at home for some patients are dysphagia (swallowing difficulties), speech impairment, and bladder and bowel disorders. Referral to the dietician, speech and language therapist, continence advisor or stoma nurse may improve quality of life for individuals dealing with complex problems resulting from their illness. However, many of these problems can lead to a negative self-image and, coupled with decreased mobility, the patient may experience boredom, decreased social skills (particularly if there are speech difficulties) and reduced social involvement. This can lead to social isolation and family strain (Turton and Orr 1993).

Case Story: Frances

Frances had developed a cancer in her mouth several years ago and had coped particularly well after the extensive surgery. She was a particularly independent lady who kept her house and garden immaculate. She went out to the shops daily and cared for her grandchildren on a regular basis. When the cancer recurred she initially dealt with this in her usual unstoppable way; however, the tumour gradually encroached further into her mouth, making speech difficult and eventually Frances was unable to swallow. She had a PEG (percutaneous

---

Case Story: Frances (*continued*)

endoscopic gastrostomy) feeding tube inserted and coped well with this. However, the family found it increasingly difficult to communicate with Frances and shopping also became a nightmare for her. She became more socially isolated and no longer found pleasure in life. As Christmas approached she seemed particularly low in mood. She told the community palliative care nurse that there was no point in spending Christmas day with the family as she could no longer communicate with them, other than through writing notes, and could not sit at the table with them for the festive meal. Shortly afterwards Frances was admitted to the local hospice where she remained until her death.

Most patients with a life-threatening illness are only too aware of the increased workload they place on family and friends. However, most will try to be as self caring as possible and keep requests for assistance to a minimum. This can be difficult when the daily household duties have to be attended to, the garden kept tidy, the car maintained and someone has to get the shopping. This will inevitably place strain on even the strongest of relationships. Add to this the practicalities of caring for the patient and it becomes apparent why there is a need for the community palliative care clinical nurse specialist and other members of the health care team, to assist these patients with not only the complex emotional problems of the illness, but also the practical problems of living at home with a life-threatening illness. However, despite these difficult problems, patients living at home are in familiar surroundings, being cared for by their family and friends, and there is more opportunity for them to have control over decision making.

During this difficult time patients may also express a need to put their affairs in order. This is a time of emotional turmoil and difficult decisions cannot be ignored or left for another time (Lee 2002). The community palliative care clinical nurse specialist can play an important role in assisting the patient with this work. These may be very emotional activities for some patients and they may require support and encouragement to achieve their goals. The activities may involve contacting or visiting old friends and family; making a will; organising their funeral; writing letters for close family members; making a memory box for children or grandchildren. The community palliative care clinical nurse specialist, in conjunction with the primary health care team, can assist patients with these and other difficulties at home in both a practical way and psychologically, to support them during their illness and in adjusting to a different life at home.

Key Points

- The losses experienced by patients with a life-threatening illness often begin from the time of diagnosis.
- The diagnosis of a life-threatening illness in one member of the family will subsequently and, sadly, affect all members of that family.
- In complex situations, where communication difficulties may have arisen, referral to the community palliative care clinical nurse specialist can be appropriate to discuss problems and facilitate the communication process between patients and their spouse or family.
- For some patients, the diagnosis of cancer and its treatments can have a marked negative effect on body image and subsequent sexuality.
- The importance of spirituality is recognised within palliative care, and helping patients to address the spiritual aspects of their lives offers the health care professional an opportunity to deliver truly holistic care.
- The community palliative care clinical nurse specialist can provide spiritual care by listening to patients, acknowledging their distress and offering them support and reassurance.
- Working alongside the other members of the primary health care team, the community palliative care clinical nurse specialist can support patients through their emotional journey and help them to regain some control over their lives.
- Not only have patients to cope with the physical, psychological, spiritual and social effects of their illness, but also they have to adapt to the practical problems that ensue as a result of their changing needs.
- The community palliative care clinical nurse specialist can provide support to the patient during this difficult time, when the individual may feel the loss of independence and increasing debility overwhelming.
- Financial considerations, due to loss of income, weigh heavily on patients who have had to give up employment due to ill health.
- The role of the community palliative care clinical nurse specialist is to empower the patient by providing information regarding state benefits and to ensure referral is made to the appropriate agencies to provide assistance.

Key Points (*continued*)

- The community palliative care clinical nurse specialist can support patients with complex psychological and practical problems and assist them to live at home with their life-threatening illness. This is achieved through collaboration with and referral to health and social work colleagues as needs arise.

Useful resources

Brennan J (2004) *Cancer in Context: A Practical Guide to Supportive Care*. Oxford University Press, Oxford.

Charlton R (ed) (2002) *Primary Palliative Care: Death, Dying and Bereavement in the Community*. Radcliffe Medical Press, Abingdon.

Cooper J (ed) (2000) *Stepping into Palliative Care: A Handbook for Community Professionals*. Radcliffe Medical Press, Abingdon.

Lloyd-Williams M (ed) (2003) *Psychosocial Issues in Palliative Care*. Oxford University Press, Oxford.

Palmer E, Howarth J (2005) *Palliative Care for the Primary Care Team*. Quay Books, London.

Payne S, Ellis-Hill C (eds) (2001) *Chronic and Terminal Illness: New Perspectives on Caring and Carers*. Oxford University Press, Oxford.

References

Altschuler J, Dale B, Byng-Hall J (1997) *Working with Chronic Illness*. Macmillan Press, Basingstoke.

Arras JD, Dubler NN (1995) Ethical and social implications of high-tech home care. In: Arras JD (ed) *Bringing the Hospital Home: Ethical and Social Implications of High-Tech Home Care*, pp 1–31. John Hopkins University Press, Baltimore.

Barnett M (2002) The development of palliative care within primary care. In: Charlton R (ed) *Primary Palliative Care: Death, Dying and Bereavement in the Community*, pp 1–14. Radcliffe Medical Press, Abingdon.

Bendall J, Muncey T (2002) Managing diabetes. In: Muncey T, Parker A (eds) (2002) *Chronic Disease Management: A Practical Guide*, pp 119–142. Palgrave, Basingstoke.

Booth R (2000) Spirituality: sharing the journey. In: Cooper J (ed) *Stepping into Palliative Care: A Handbook for Community Professionals*, pp 127–135. Radcliffe Medical Press, Abingdon.

Bowling A (1995) *Measuring Disease*. Open University Press, Buckingham.

Brennan J (2004) *Cancer in Context: A Practical Guide to Supportive Care*. Oxford University Press, Oxford.

Burton M, Watson M (1998) *Counselling People with Cancer*. Wiley and Sons, Chichester.

Carr AJ, Gibson B, Robinson PG (2001) Is quality of life determined by expectations or experience? *British Medical Journal* 322, 1240–1243.

Clark B (2002) Spirituality and ethnicity. In: Charlton R (ed) *Primary Palliative Care: Death, Dying and Bereavement in the Community*, pp 155–163. Radcliffe Medical Press, Abingdon.

Cooper GM (1993) *The Cancer Book*. Jones and Bartlett, Boston.

Coote A (1996) Options for long-term care. In: Harding T, Meredith B, Wistow G (eds) *Options for Long-Term Care*, pp 99–106. HMSO, London.

Crumbie A (2002) Patient–professional relationships. In: Crumbie A, Lawrence J (eds) *Living with a Chronic Condition: A Practitioner's Guide to Providing Care*, pp 3–15. Butterworth Heinemann, Oxford.

Curtin M, Lubkin I (1998) What is chronicity. In: Lubkin IM, Larsen PD (eds) *Chronic Illness: Impact and Interventions*, 4th edn, pp 3–25. Jones and Bartlett, Sudbury.

Davy J, Ellis S (2000) *Counselling Skills in Palliative Care*. Open University Press, Buckingham.

Deegan P (1996) Recovery as a journey of the heart. *Psychiatric Rehabilitation Journal* 19 (3), 91–97.

Department of Health (2001) *The Expert Patient: A New Approach to Chronic Disease Management for the 21st Century*. HMSO, London.

Doyle D, Jeffrey D (2000) *Palliative Care in the Home*. Oxford University Press, Oxford.

Dryden H (2003) Body image. In: Faithful S, Wells M (eds) *Supportive Care in Radiotherapy*, pp 320—336. Churchill Livingstone, Edinburgh.

Gerardi R (1989) Western spirituality and health care. In: Carson VB *Spiritual Dimensions of Nursing Practice*, pp 76–112. WB Saunders, London.

Hasler J (1990) The size and nature of the problem. In: Hasler J, Schofield T (eds) (1990) *Continuing Care: The Management of Chronic Disease*, 2nd edn, pp 13–16. Oxford Medical Publications, Oxford.

Hermann CP (2001) Spiritual needs of dying patients: a qualitative study. *Oncology Nursing Forum* 28 (1), 67–72.

Hunt J, Cobb M, Keeley VL, Ahmedzai SH (2003) The quality of spiritual care – developing a standard. *International Journal of Palliative Nursing* 9 (5), 208–214.

Hurdman R (1995) Meeting social needs – the role of the social worker. In: Robbins J, Moscrop J (eds) *Caring for the Dying Patient and the Family*, 3rd edn, pp 115–124. Chapman and Hall, London.

Kelly M (1992) Self identity and radical surgery. *Sociology of Health and Illness* 14 (3), 390–415.

Kemp C (1999) *Terminal Illness: A Guide to Nursing Care*, 2nd edn. Lippincott, Philadelphia.

Larsen PD, Kahn AM, Flodberg SO (1998) Sexuality. In: Lubkin IM, Larsen PD (eds) *Chronic Illness: Impact and Interventions*, 4th edn, pp 299–323. Jones and Bartlett, Sudbury.

Lee E (2002) *In Your Own Time: A Guide for Patients and Their Carers Facing a Last Illness at Home*. Oxford University Press, Oxford.

McKenzie H, Boughton M, Hayes L, et al. (2007) A sense of security for cancer patients at home: the role of community nurses. *Health and Social Care in the Community* 15 (4), 352–359.

McMurray A (2004) Older people. In: Oliviere D, Monroe B (eds) *Death, Dying and Social Differences*, pp 63–77. Oxford University Press, Oxford.

Monroe B, Sheldon F (2004) Psychosocial dimensions of care. In: Sykes N, Edmonds P, Wiles J (eds) *Management of Advanced Disease*, 4th edn, pp 405–437. Arnold, London.

Oliver D (2000) The special needs of the neurological patient. In: Cooper J (ed) *Stepping into Palliative Care: A Handbook for Community Professionals*, pp 223–234. Radcliffe Medical Press, Abingdon.

O'Neill J, Leedham K (2001) Rehabilitation and long term effects of treatment. In: Corner J, Bailey C (eds) *Cancer Nursing: Care in Context*, pp 442–448. Blackwell Science, Oxford.

Palmer E, Howarth J (2005) *Palliative Care for the Primary Care Team*. Quay Books, London.

Payne S, Ellis-Hill C (2001) Being a carer. In: Payne S, Ellis-Hill C (eds) *Chronic and Terminal Illness: New Perspectives on Caring and Carers*, pp 1–21. Oxford University Press, Oxford.

Plant H (2001) The impact of cancer on the family. In: Corner J, Bailey C (eds) *Cancer Nursing: Care in Context*, pp 86–99. Blackwell Science, Oxford.

Radley A (1994) *Making Sense of Illness: The Social Psychology of Health and Disease*. Sage, London.

Rose K (2001) A longitudinal study of carers providing palliative care. In: Payne S, Ellis-Hill C (eds) *Chronic and Terminal Illness: New*

Perspectives on Caring and Carers, pp 64–82. Oxford University Press, Oxford.

Ross L (1994) Spiritual care: the nurse's role. *Nursing Standard* 8 (29), 33–37.

Sheldon F (2003) Social impact of advanced metastatic cancer. In: Lloyd-Williams M (ed) *Psychosocial Issues in Palliative Care*, pp 35–48. Oxford University Press, Oxford.

Speck PW (2004) Spiritual concerns. In: Sykes N, Edmonds P, Wiles J (eds) *Management of Advanced Disease*, 4th edn, pp 471–481. Arnold, London.

Stoll RI (1989) Spirituality in chronic illness. In: Carson VB (ed) *Spiritual Dimensions of Nursing Practice*, pp 180–216. WB Saunders, London.

Strauss AL, Corbin J, Fagerhaugh S, et al. (1984) *Chronic Illness and the Quality of Life*, 2nd edn. Mosby, London.

Turton P, Orr J (1993) *Learning to Care in the Community*, 2nd edn. Edward Arnold, London.

White N, Richter J, Fry C (1992) Coping, social support and adaptation to chronic illness. *Western Journal of Nursing Research* 14 (2), 211–224.

Whyte DA (ed) (1997) *Explorations of Family Nursing*. Routledge, London.

Wilkie P (1998) The person, the patient and their carers. In: Faull C, Carter Y, Woof R (eds) *Handbook of Palliative Care*, pp 55–63. Blackwell Science, Oxford.

Woof R, Nyatanga B (1998) Adapting to death, dying and bereavement. In: Faull C, Carter Y, Woof R (eds) *Handbook of Palliative Care*, pp 74–87. Blackwell Science, Oxford.

Woof R, Carter Y, Faull C (1998) Palliative care: the team, the services and the need for care. In: Faull C, Carter Y, Woof R (eds) *Handbook of Palliative Care*, pp 13–32. Blackwell Science, Oxford.

Dying at Home: The Emotional Journey

Introduction

Nursing care of patients who are dying has undergone considerable change in the last 40 years since the emergence of the hospice movement. Palliative care is now well established in the United Kingdom and aims to relieve the physical, psychological, social and spiritual needs of patients approaching the end of their life. Dying and death are a natural part of life; however, people differ in their response to the prospect of death, and many are faced with problems that are too painful to discuss and/or resolve. Leaving behind a partner, children, siblings and parents can be difficult issues to work through. Being at home, however, allows patients a greater opportunity to determine their own care, and receiving information about end of life care, discussing complex emotions and communicating with the family are all sensitive issues which the community palliative care clinical nurse specialist can address with the patient. No individual can meet all the needs of the patient approaching death and therefore multidisciplinary teamwork lies at the heart of effective palliative care in the home, where the community palliative care clinical nurse specialist works alongside the other members of the primary health care team to deliver a service tailored to the wishes of the dying patient.

The team approach

As demonstrated in previous chapters, the role of the community palliative care clinical nurse specialist, as part of the specialist palliative care services, is varied and complex. For patients nearing the end of life, referral to the community palliative care clinical nurse specialist is usually instigated by the primary health care team or hospital palliative care team. Reasons for referral may include advice on pain and symptom control, especially where there are numerous symptoms, psychosocial or spiritual distress, complicated family issues or complex end of life problems. The community palliative care clinical nurse specialist may be directly involved with patients and their families or may be indirectly involved through the primary health care team. The indirect role will include guiding and/or advising colleagues on a variety of issues which may encompass ongoing symptom control, advice about research or best practice, encouraging reflective practice, facilitating significant event analysis, or supporting colleagues in complex case management.

The Royal College of Nursing in the United Kingdom (2002) set out recommended core competencies for specialist nursing in palliative care. These competencies include communication, quality assurance, clinical practice, education, management and leadership, research and development and grief, loss and bereavement. The direct and indirect services that the community palliative care clinical nurse specialist has to offer will include a balance of clinical experience and competency, as well as academic and theoretical knowledge. Through collaboration with other members of the primary health care team, the community palliative care clinical nurse specialist aims to deliver high-quality care to those patients nearing the end of life. The team may be utilising a tool such as the Gold Standards Framework to facilitate improved coordination, communication and delivery of palliative care to the patient (Thomas 2003). This tool is supported by Macmillan Cancer Support and has been rolled out to many areas within the United Kingdom.

The multidisciplinary members of the primary health care team all have their role in the care of the dying patient at home. However, the district nurse is usually the key professional involved in the day-to-day practical nursing care of the patient. Caring for the dying patient is primarily a nursing responsibility and the district nurse and community palliative care clinical nurse specialist will work together to meet the needs of the patient, and at times this may result in a blurring of the roles. To deliver holistic care the district nurse will also be involved in symptom control and emotional support, whilst the community palliative care clinical nurse specialist may, at times, have to organise equipment or give advice on practical problems. The district nurse will look to the community palliative care clinical nurse specialist for advice on a variety of complex problems, such as pain and symptom control.

Research has demonstrated that district nurses experience difficulties when dealing with patients' symptoms, and a study by Dunne et al. (2005) identified pain as the single most complex symptom for the district nurse to contend with during the palliative stages of a patient's illness. The role of the community palliative care clinical nurse specialist is to assist the district nurse and other members of the primary health care team with complex problems and together ensure that the patient is comfortable and confident to remain in his or her own home until death.

The role of the community palliative care clinical nurse specialist is also to provide support and information to patients nearing the end of life; this may involve listening, talking, reassurance, help or advice. According to Lee (2002), it is the gift of time that enables community palliative care clinical nurse specialists to provide effective care of patients, as they have time to sit and listen to patients and are trained to *hear* what the patient is saying. Indirectly, they are often working behind the scenes in coordinating care and also offering specialist advice to general practitioners and district nurses (Payne et al. 2004). Many patients will present with complex circumstances and distressing symptoms; these difficult situations are challenging to all the health professionals involved; however, effective end of life care can be delivered through anticipating problems, minimising crisis and working together to support patients in their last weeks or days of life.

End of life care

In today's society the decision to be cared for and die at home is not an easy one, for a variety of reasons. Although figures suggest that around three quarters of terminally ill patients express a wish to die at home, currently only about a quarter of them actually do so (Lakasing and Mahaffey 2006). Patients will have their fears about the dying process, anxieties concerning pain and other symptoms at the end of life, how they will react to approaching death and whether their family will be able to care for them until the end.

Caring for patients who are dying has always been part of the everyday work of health professionals and the aim is to achieve the optimum quality of life for the patient. The important aspects of caring for the dying are listening, allowing the individual to retain control, and providing optimum physical and emotional comfort (Wells 2001). Patients and their families will look towards the health professionals to support them in a *good* death. This usually means that patients' physical symptoms have been well controlled, they have had time to say good-bye to family and friends, they feel well supported emotionally and they have also been able to face death with dignity (Wong et al. 2004). This journey may last weeks or days and may well be fraught with problems. However, many of the fears about death can be overcome through information and support, allowing the patient to die in familiar surroundings with loved ones in attendance.

Case Story: Archie

Archie knew his life was drawing to a close. Unfortunately he had been admitted into the local hospital by the out-of-hours doctor on a Saturday evening. He had experienced an episode of acute breathlessness and his wife had felt unable to deal with his symptoms. Archie wanted to die at home and his wife was aware of his wishes. The community palliative care clinical nurse specialist spoke to Archie's wife on the Monday morning and she accepted the help of Marie Curie nurses for overnight monitoring, to allow Archie to come home. Explanation was given on how to manage Archie's breathlessness and other symptoms. She was reassured that help was only a telephone call away. Archie came home on the Monday afternoon and died peacefully 2 days later with his wife and daughters present.

One important aspect in the care of patients who are facing death is to allow patients to remain in control of their situation for as long as possible. However, to exercise autonomy dying individuals must be fully informed about what is happening to them and able to make choices regarding their care. They may wish to express their preferences regarding place of death, the level of care and support they want from the professionals or their family, use of particular medications (in accordance with cultural or religious beliefs) or indeed whom they want to know about their situation. The community palliative care clinical nurse specialist may be involved with patients to give information, assist them in their options and ensure that their wishes are made known to other members of the health care team. Dying individuals are most likely to be worried about being abandoned, losing control over their own bodies or being in pain and distress (Corr et al. 2003). The majority of patients will value open and sensitive discussion about their impending death; however, the health professional must take into account the fear that the prospect of death invokes and therefore impart information only when requested by the patient. As the disease progresses and death approaches, the needs and wishes of the patient may change and it is necessary to continually reassess the situation with the individual to ensure his or her continuing needs are being met. To help patients achieve what they want requires a needs-led approach to care which does not restrict patients in their preferred choices (Sheldon 1997).

Emotions and feelings facing death

When patients are diagnosed with a life-threatening illness they face the inevitability of death at some point in the future. However, after months or perhaps years of ill health, the news that the illness has progressed and death is approaching still comes as a shock to the patient. Emotions such as anger, anxiety and fear are common. Anger, for example, can be directed at the medical or nursing staff and patients may require the opportunity to discuss their feelings with the person or persons at whom the anger is directed. The anger is at times an expression of feeling overwhelmed or frightened and may be appropriate to the situation. Dealing with an angry patient can be a daunting prospect and the health professional needs to try to understand the cause of the anger in order to diffuse it (Kilbler 1996). Sometimes anger is targeted towards the family and they will need considerable support and explanation to understand this situation (Bycroft and Brown 1996); however, if the anger is directed at staff, family or carers, it can alienate those who want to give care and support (Twycross 1999).

According to Fisher (2002), anger is a powerful emotion and if patients are unable to vent their feelings, they can become depressed and cut themselves off from others. Patients will need time and space to express their anger, which may result from their feelings of powerlessness and a desire to regain some control of their world (Sheldon 2004). However, it should be remembered that symptoms such as fatigue or breathlessness may make it more difficult for patients to communicate strong emotions and they may require alternative methods, such as pen and paper, to report what they are feeling. Unfortunately some patients never resolve their anger before death approaches.

Case Story: Sharon

Sharon was 54 years old. She was diagnosed with advanced cancer just after gaining promotion at work. She had attributed her symptoms initially to the pressures of her employment and the stress of

---

Case Story: Sharon (*continued*)

working for the promotion. Sharon's condition deteriorated rapidly and it was soon evident that she would be unable to return to the job she had worked so hard to gain. Sharon became angry with everyone: family, friends and especially the health care professionals. She expressed her anger by shouting, screaming and, at times, locking the door to everyone. The general practitioner asked the community palliative care clinical nurse specialist to visit Sharon and assist the team in dealing with Sharon's anger. Sharon was angry at life, at the disease itself and at the professionals for failing to 'cure' her of the disease. She was allowed to express her feelings, but sadly died before she could resolve her anger or accept her situation.

Life-threatening illness creates an uncertain future and this causes anxiety, which may increase as the illness progresses (Regnard and Tempest 1998) and death approaches. Anxiety is found in about a quarter of patients nearing the end of life (Barraclough 1999) and is a normal response to unfamiliar or unpredictable situations (Furlong and O'Toole 2006). The anxiety may result from their concerns about the unknown, how they will die, death itself and what lies thereafter. The anxiety may manifest in physical symptoms such as nausea or diarrhoea, sweating or dry mouth, or the patient may complain of sleeping badly or having frightening dreams (Twycross 1999). If anxiety escalates the patient will become increasingly distracted from daily activities and unable to make everyday decisions. Anxiety symptoms are distressing and debilitating in their own right and may result in frightening panic attacks (Henderson 2004). This can result in the patient being afraid to be alone and expressing a need for a friend or family member to be close at all times. This can be very difficult for family members to sustain and may result in carer fatigue. Recognising anxiety in patients and allowing them to talk about it is an important part of management (Barraclough 1999).

Case Story: Jeremy

Jeremy was nearing death, but the district nurses reported he seemed anxious and restless at times. His wife was concerned about this and asked for the community palliative care clinical nurse specialist to talk to him. He reported that his affairs were all in order and he had said his goodbyes, but now that death was closer he began to be anxious about what awaited him after death. He had been afraid to divulge this to others, as he may have appeared to have lost his faith in God. The community palliative care clinical nurse specialist, with Jeremy's permission, contacted the minister from the local church and he visited Jeremy. He found great comfort in his visit and became more settled. He died peacefully 3 days later.

Anxiety is a complex problem that is often confused with fear. Patients need to be aware that to feel fear and experience anxiety is part of the adjustment process to impending death and that they will need time with health care professionals, like the community palliative care clinical nurse specialist, to explore their feelings (Jeffrey 2000). Like other emotions, fear can be expressed in words or in behaviour. If patients can be assisted to recognise their fears and talk about them, it may help to gain some control over the situation. The community palliative care clinical nurse specialist can provide time and expertise to assist patients in expressing their fears. This may take time and several visits for patients to feel comfortable and start to express their innermost emotions. Common fears are of the symptoms associated with death, the death itself or what happens after death. There may also be specific fears such as bleeding or choking to death, which may or may not be well founded (Barraclough 1999). Patients may be helped to overcome their fears through accurate information about the dying process, being given time to express their fears, and reassurance that medical and nursing assistance is available, during the day and night, should difficulties arise at home.

Case Story: Grace

Grace had an aggressive oral cancer and her condition was deteriorating. The community nurses reported that she had become agitated and very weepy. They asked the community palliative care clinical nurse specialist to visit Grace to try to determine the problem. Initially Grace was reluctant to express her concerns, but gradually she revealed that she had a great fear of choking to death. She was sure that the tumour would obstruct her airway. Grace required information and careful explanation about the dying process. She was relieved to hear that she was unlikely to die in a sudden choking event. Grace died very quietly and peacefully at home a few weeks later.

For many patients, facing death is their greatest challenge (Kemp 1999); however, death is an inevitable part of life. Individuals who are dying still have a broad range of needs and desires, hopes, fears and anxieties (Corr et al. 2003). All patients reach their time of dying with differing life experiences, different cultural responses and with their own psychological and spiritual issues. Each dying patient is unique and reactions to impending death will be unique to the individual. As life nears its end, the quality of life that is left becomes a major concern for patients, their families and the health professionals. Quality of life is a key component of palliative care and it is important for the health professional visiting the dying patient at home to understand what quality of life means to that patient and ensure goals and needs are being realised. Quality of life is a term that can refer to an individual's physical, emotional, social and spiritual well-being and may be achieved through promoting autonomy and choice, good symptom relief and listening to the patient (Mirando 2006). However, many other factors may influence quality of life for dying patients, including relationships with their family and friends, feeling secure and looked after, being in the place of their choosing and their involvement in life at home.

Family and social support

Relationships with family and friends are important to most people, but in today's society families are becoming ever more complex. There are more lone-parent families, same-sex couples and many extended families now live considerable distances from the *family* home. However, when faced with a crisis or uncertainty, most individuals depend on their family and friends for support, protection and security. Where patients lack support they become more vulnerable to the emotional effects of their illness, notably anxiety and depression (Brennan 2004).

Family dynamics will inevitably vary from one household to another and it is important for the health professionals to develop an understanding of each patient's family and their reaction to the patient's illness and impending death. When assessing the patient, it is essential to gain an insight into how the family functions, the conflicts, the supportive members and the vulnerable individuals (Jeffrey 2003). The patient's role within the family is also important and the many changes that his or her illness has inflicted on that role. Whilst dealing with the changes, family members may have to adapt and respond to a change in their own roles, causing significant stress to individual members (McIntyre and Lugton 2005).

However, for many patients this is a time for looking back over their life and perhaps for resolving conflicts or re-establishing contact with family and friends who have become estranged. For some patients, talking with their family and friends will give them the opportunity to discuss past events, give meaning to their contribution within the family and relive happy occasions. Allowing patients to talk and express their feelings and thoughts can enable them to feel more in control of events (Brennan 2004). However, for individuals who are socially isolated or lack family support, the community palliative care clinical nurse specialist may be the professional who offers the time, to allow the patient to talk.

As well as being a source of support, family and friends may be a source of stress to the patient. Support from other family members may not always be as patients had expected; those they regarded as *reliable* in a crisis may find the situation too distressing and need support themselves. The patient's family may be anxious, distraught and saddened at the prospect of losing a loved one. As a result, the patient may be the one providing ongoing support to the family. This may not allow individual patients to deal with their own emotions and they may feel guilty for the distress they are causing to others. They therefore need the opportunity to express their own feelings, and the health professionals involved with the patient have to recognise this need. Referral to the community palliative care clinical nurse specialist would be appropriate, to allow patients time and the opportunity to deal with their own complex anxieties, fears and concerns. Patients' relationships are complex because of the past life that has shaped the individual, and at times the patient may feel the need or desire to confide and discuss difficult issues or concerns (Brennan 2004).

Case Story: Rosemary

Rosemary was a retired lady of 75 years of age who had a very caring husband and family. One day she asked to speak to the community palliative care clinical nurse specialist alone. Rosemary had something she wanted to talk about, but knew it would cause her husband and family distress. She then proceeded to relate a distressing story of physical and sexual abuse that she had suffered whilst a child. No living person knew about the abuse and she had never confided it to anyone before. The role of the community palliative care clinical nurse specialist was to listen and acknowledge what Rosemary was relating and allow her to vent her deep-rooted emotions. Rosemary became very upset and tearful but thanked the nurse for listening. Rosemary had needed to tell someone about this before she died.

At times it can be difficult for patients to express their emotions, anxieties and fears to their family and relatives, because of a need to protect them from further distress. This protection may also derive from a sense of shielding their loved ones from subjects that are uncomfortable or embarrassing to talk about. At times, this may result in both patient and family feeling increasingly estranged by their inability to talk freely and openly with one another (Johnston 2004). However, as identified above, sometimes patients have a need to verbalise issues that are too distressing to discuss with family members and require the assistance of a health professional, such as the community palliative care clinical nurse specialist, to *hear* their problems.

Social support is one of the most important resources that most patients have in coping with the stress of dying. That support may be from family, friends or good neighbours. They need to be able to talk through their problems and express their feelings. However, health care staff should be aware that although patients may appear to have good support systems, the individuals may not be perceived by the patient as supportive. This may be due to a variety of reasons, such as cultural differences, being too distressed to be supportive or perhaps the patient does not want to appear a *burden* on others by relating his/her concerns and anxieties. Therefore, access to additional emotional support is essential for all those who desire it (Brennan 2004). Referral to the community palliative care clinical nurse specialist should be considered by the primary health care team, in order to allow patients the opportunity to express their concerns and anxieties. Explanation may be necessary for patients to feel comfortable expressing their feelings; they need to be informed that it is very natural to have complex emotions when faced with impending death.

Communicating within the family

For many patients the need to express their feelings and communicate their emotions can be particularly difficult. The skilled community palliative care clinical nurse specialist can help with this process, however, for some patients difficulties arise when trying to communicate with their loved ones. They may feel uncomfortable attempting to express emotions, embarrassed at trying to relay how they feel or anxious about creating more upset and distress to their family at this difficult time. Patients may want to say final goodbyes, tell their family how much they are loved or leave instructions about the future. At times it will be necessary for the community palliative care clinical nurse specialist to act as facilitator in these situations, to encourage open communication and offer support to patients and their families.

Complicated scenarios can arise when the patient and family do not speak about the illness or the impending death, but instead choose to act as though nothing is wrong (Doyle and Jeffrey 2000). This can be counter-productive for patients who want to put their affairs in order, perhaps make preparations for the family's future or heal broken relationships from the past. Many families never talk about what really matters and therefore it can be particularly difficult to start meaningful communication when someone is dying. A sensitive approach by the community palliative care clinical nurse specialist can assist the patient to open dialogue with the family and start communication around distressing topics. The age, gender, stage in life and culture can also affect the communication process and the patient's ability to reveal emotions and discuss his or her own death. Discussing death makes it very real and causes considerable distress; however, ignoring the inevitable leaves patients and their families feeling isolated and unable to express their fears and sadness (Brennan 2004).

Case Story: Catherine

Catherine had been suffering from bowel cancer for 8 years. She had had chemotherapy on numerous occasions and radiotherapy for spinal metastases. She had kept remarkably well during her illness and had never verbalised with her husband or family that the cancer would one day lead to her death. In fact she had always trivialised the seriousness of the illness, believing that this would cause the family less distress. Persistent mild pains in her abdomen and back were always related to minor complaints, such as too much gardening or something she had eaten. When pain became an increasing problem and scans revealed further spinal activity, Catherine was informed that the illness was progressing and treatment options were now more limited. The oncologist caring for Catherine asked the community palliative care clinical nurse specialist to visit Catherine to discuss relaying the seriousness of the situation to her family. Catherine admitted that she was aware of what was happening, but would not consider talking to her husband or family about death. She refused to allow the community palliative care clinical nurse specialist to intervene, believing that she knew her family best. After Catherine's death, her husband had a very distressing and difficult time coming to terms with the silence and pretence they had endured over many years and particularly in the months leading to her death. He required bereavement counselling for many months.

It can be particularly sad when a family does not communicate, often on the basis that they are protecting each other, and ultimately never speaks about the important things that matter to the individual (Neuberger 2004). However, not only is it difficult for patients to discuss issues with their spouse and other adult family members, but also it can be particularly challenging and distressing when children have to be told to prepare themselves for the death of a parent. The pain of leaving children is so overwhelming that sometimes parents cannot face talking to their children about what is happening (Lee 2002). Patients often turn to the health professionals for guidance on how best to relay the news to their children. The community palliative care clinical nurse specialist can offer assistance to patients at this distressing time, giving reassurance, advice and offering to include the children in discussions.

Communicating with children

Health care professionals often assume that families will communicate with children when a parent or close family member is dying. However, at times the family will require help with this daunting task; the help may simply be sitting, listening and being with a family as they impart the bad news (Jeffrey 1998). Most children will report that regardless of whether they are told or not, they know that something is wrong. When they see their mother, father or other close relative upset and crying, they instinctively know something is very wrong. Children need and should be given the same honest information imparted to adults. The only difference is that the information requires to be tailored to the age and understanding of the child. The child also requires time to comprehend what has been said and sometime later should be given the opportunity to ask further questions.

It is important that children are not excluded from what is happening, and many will report having overheard telephone calls, noticed someone in tears or have wondered why the doctor or nurse was visiting so frequently. Parents will naturally want to protect their children from any pain or distress; however. saying nothing will add to the child's confusion and fear. Parents need to be helped to see how impossible it is to keep the situation from their children and the community palliative care clinical nurse specialist can assist with this difficult task.

Case Story: Gregory

Gregory was only 41 years old. He had two daughters aged 7 and 9 years. He was admitted to hospital after a collapse and found to have bleeding brain metastases from a metastatic malignant melanoma. The doctor told his wife that he may not survive the night. His wife had the difficult task of preparing the girls for the death of their father. She managed this with the help of her own parents. However, Gregory survived and eventually made it home. He had reduced mobility and other physical problems but managed to participate in family life for a further 2 months. He then started to deteriorate and it became obvious that he was dying. His wife was completely unable to tell the girls again that their father was dying; she had been through this scenario once before and could not do it again. The community palliative care clinical nurse specialist visited the house and, with the assistance of their mother, told the girls that their father was dying and not going to recover as he had before. The girls were upset but reported seeing changes in their father and realised that he must be ill again. They were glad someone had spoken to them and asked if they could help to look after their dad.

A key role of the community palliative care clinical nurse specialist is to assist parents to inform their children and help to prepare them for the difficulties ahead (Sheldon 1997). Many children use play to communicate their feelings and thoughts and may require games or drawings to allow them the opportunity to express themselves. Encouraging children to write short stories may also assist them to communicate their fears and concerns. At times, it may be helpful for the community palliative care clinical nurse specialist to refer to a social worker, asking the social worker to visit the family and help the parents and children with these difficult issues and prepare them for the future.

Children tend to be overprotected from the impact of serious illness and impending death; this will be done in order to protect the child or children, but can create problems. The children may be left with feelings of anger or sadness, they may feel that their opportunity to say goodbye was denied, or that they were excluded and left feeling isolated from the whole situation (Palmer and Howarth 2005). Children should be included in open discussion about what is happening. The role of the community palliative care clinical nurse specialist is to work with parents, supporting them and encouraging them to talk with their children. Children, just as adults, all react differently to distressing situations and it may be important to encourage the familiar family and household routines, or enlist the help of grandparents or other family members to offer support to the children. Some children, depending on their age and understanding, may wish to help care for their dying parent; this may give the child precious time with the parent and an opportunity to talk. This also allows the child to become familiar with the appearance, frailty and weakness of the dying parent. Each child is different and his or her response to what is happening will be different; the community palliative care clinical nurse specialist can assist and support parents to communicate with their children, reassuring them that their children will be better prepared for the death, if they are aware of what is happening.

Around the death

Not only is it necessary to prepare children for death, but also many adults have never witnessed the death of a close relative or friend. As death at home is less frequent in today's society, few family members will have had any previous experience in caring for an individual who is dying. This can make the dying process all the more frightening to patients and their close families. Images of death and dying created on television and cinema screens do not add up to the reality of what may be happening within a patient's home and the complexity of feelings and overwhelming emotions being experienced by the patient and family. Sensitive communication between patients, their families and the health professionals is needed to allow the patients to make decisions and choices regarding their care and for families to feel well supported in caring for their loved one, until the time of death. For those patients who have chosen to remain at home, it is useful for health professionals, such as the community palliative care clinical nurse specialist, to talk about the time of death before it is imminent, to provide accurate information about the dying process, acknowledge fears and ensure that the patient feels the level of support being given is adequate (Sheldon 1997).

Strategies to support patients and carers

During the difficult weeks and days leading to a patient's death, the level of support required may vary, depending on the general condition of the patient. At times, as discussed in the previous chapter, the family routine can become totally absorbed in fulfilling hospital and clinic appointments, health care professionals' visits and attendance at a variety of other illness-related appointments. However, as the illness trajectory moves on and the general condition of the patient deteriorates, it is important to ensure that all unnecessary appointments are cancelled and that the health care professionals visiting the home are made aware of the changes in the patient. The community palliative care clinical nurse specialist can negotiate with the patient, in a sensitive manner, which appointments or health care professionals may be cancelled. It would be inappropriate to expect a patient to travel considerable distance, using up valuable energy resources, to attend a clinic appointment which will achieve no beneficial outcome for the dying patient.

The patient may also feel overwhelmed by the number of health and social care professionals visiting the home, and again careful negotiation with patients, their families and the professionals involved may be able to reduce the numbers to a level more acceptable to patients. This again allows patients to take control of the situation, with regard to the frequency and timing of home visits, and allows them to save their energy for the things they value most at this time (Proot et al. 2004). This may be a fine balancing act between ensuring adequate services are being provided to support patients and families, and allowing them privacy and control over the situation. The last few weeks or days of a patient's life are a *special* time, no matter how difficult, and overly enthusiastic professionals may have to be urged to decrease visiting to allow quality time for the patient and loved ones.

This quality time may also extend to curtailing visits and telephone calls from well-meaning family and friends. Many patients find visitors very tiring and often report they feel completely exhausted after visitors leave the house. Not wanting to seem ungrateful, many patients tolerate these visits, reporting later that they are unable to enjoy the company, because of fatigue and other related symptoms. They may also experience feelings of guilt for seeming reluctant to have visitors, when they know people are trying to be kind and supportive. However, these visits may also impinge on the quality time and privacy they may desire with their own spouse or partner, or indeed with their children.

It may be necessary for the community palliative care clinical nurse specialist to explain to the patient that these complex feelings are normal in this situation and explore with the patient strategies to deal with the problem. This may be simple methods such as allowing telephone calls to go onto an answering machine, or asking individuals only to call at designated times. Visitors can be asked to restrict the length of their visits to a specified time, perhaps 20–30 minutes, and only visit at certain times of the day. However, it may even be necessary to put a notice on the front door asking visitors not to disturb at particular times, or not to ring the doorbell when the patient is resting. These simple methods can often make life more tolerable for patients and their families; however, until voiced by the patient and acknowledged by the community palliative care clinical nurse specialist, these problems may have seemed insurmountable.

Case Story: John

John and his wife had both been married before and had large extended families who all visited frequently. They lived in a little village where neighbours rallied round to help others in times of trouble. Life had been very busy, with the house full of guests most weekends and social events most evenings. John was now very ill with pancreatic cancer and had expressed a wish to die at home. Initially the support offered from family, friends and neighbours was gratefully appreciated and his wife found great comfort knowing that someone was always visiting. However, this was now becoming difficult to control, with little time for John and his wife to be alone. John was becoming increasingly anxious about the situation and wanted everyone to go away and leave them in peace. His wife asked the community palliative care clinical nurse specialist for help and advice on how to deal with the situation. Initially simple measures such as restricting times of telephone calls and visiting periods worked well, but as his condition further deteriorated the calls and visitors again started to increase. The community palliative care clinical nurse specialist assisted John and his wife to make a list of those whom John would want visiting the house, for example close family, and all others were to be informed politely that John was too tired to receive visitors. His wife agreed to contact other friends and neighbours by telephone to keep them updated; this she could do when John was resting, thereby reducing the number of telephone calls into the house. John was very happy with this resolution and found he could again relax and enjoy peace and privacy with his wife.

For patients facing death, having autonomy and retaining some control over their situation is increasingly important, particularly as they deal with losses in their physical function. This may be difficult for patients, as their growing weakness is a constant reminder of the advancing disease and their lack of control over the illness. Initially patients may find the stairs a problem, then walking on the level becomes more difficult and one day they realise assistance is required to transfer to the toilet. As the weakness progresses, patients may need to use a commode, may be confined to the chair most of the day and gradually they spend more time in bed. Adjustment to these losses can be particularly difficult, as the patient becomes aware that the deterioration is now progressive and more evident to others. Patients will require the opportunity to express their sadness, frustration and anger as the illness takes its toll on their daily life. The community palliative care clinical nurse specialist can explore with patients their complex emotions and try to develop simple strategies to allow the patient, although less mobile, to still participate in family life within the home. Husbands may still need to be involved in decisions regarding finance; mothers will still want to care for their children, however limited their physical resources; and the elderly will still have a need to be involved in their family's lives.

Case Story: Molly

Molly was living with her daughter and grandchildren; life in her own home had become more difficult due to her increasing weakness. She enjoyed the noise in her daughter's house and hearing the voices of her grandchildren at play. They still came into her room to ask for help with schoolwork and have little chats with her. Molly still felt part of their lives and, despite her rapidly advancing illness, allowed the grandchildren to help her in little ways. The community palliative care clinical nurse specialist listened to Molly express her sadness at leaving the family; however, Molly managed to retain some control over her care and also involved the grandchildren where possible, even if it was only to bring her a drink. Despite her frailty she participated in family life, albeit limited, until the end of her own life. She died very peacefully with her daughter and grandchildren around the bed.

Care of the older patient

Careful assessment and knowledge of the patient's wishes are essential requirements in planning care for the older patient. However, older patients with a life-threatening illness may also have to contend with other age-related chronic conditions such as arthritis, hypertension, diabetes, dementia and cardiovascular problems, all of which may have taken their toll on the older person's general health, prior to the onset of their present illness. Add to this their possible difficulties with hearing and visual impairments, general frailty and reduced ability to perform the daily activities of living (cooking, cleaning, self-care, etc.) and it is clearly evident that the older patient may require considerable support during their final illness. Brennan (2004) also reports that older patients may be reluctant to report their difficulties, be they physical (e.g. pain), social (e.g. isolation) or emotional distress (e.g. depression). The role of the community palliative care clinical nurse, in conjunction with the primary health care team, is to offer support to these older patients and give them an opportunity to express their emotions, discuss their symptoms and assess where help of a practical nature is required.

Older patients may also be concerned about the effects of their illness on the elderly spouse who may be caring for them (Wilkie 1998). This creates a unique situation where the spouse, as well as the patient, may be in need of practical care and support. The community palliative care clinical nurse specialist can provide information to the elderly couple regarding care options and offer reassurance that their wishes will be taken into consideration. As mentioned previously, many elderly are quite isolated as extended families no longer live in close proximity, and changing demographics show that as people grow older in today's society, more of them live on their own (Brennan 2004). This can result in isolation and loneliness for many elderly patients. The community palliative care clinical nurse specialist can offer time and expertise to elderly patients, ensuring that their needs are addressed and their preferred place of death is made known to the other members of the health care team. Death remains just as fearful to the older person as it is to the younger patient, and although more support may be necessary, the elderly can achieve their wish to die at home if desired.

Culture and religion

Whilst addressing the palliative care needs of any dying patient, be they elderly or at an earlier stage in their life, the health care professional also requires to be sensitive to the cultural practices and customs of patients and their families. The concept of culture includes the values, beliefs, morals, traditions and language of a particular group and may incorporate ethnic origin and religion (Kemp 1999). Culture can be described as *rules* or *guidelines* which individuals inherit or acquire as members of a particular society and which instructs them how to view the world (Sheldon 1997). Attitudes to sickness, life and death are also culturally determined and may have a bearing on how people behave and respond to others. Closely linked to culture are spiritual and religious beliefs and they may have an influence on how patients interpret their illness (Lloyd-Williams 2003).

The diagnosis of a life-threatening illness and the knowledge that death is approaching is a source of considerable distress and suffering to all concerned; however, a patient's response to that knowledge may be affected by his or her culture, beliefs and religion. This may have the potential for misunderstandings and difficulties between the patient and health care professionals. However, nurses working in the community are often more familiar with the cultural and religious variations in families because they visit individuals in their own homes (Neuberger 2004). The community palliative care clinical nurse specialist will also have knowledge of the various cultural beliefs and religious practices encountered within the community and the diverse cultural rituals affiliated with death. Many of these will be associated with particular religious groups, and in today's multicultural and multifaith society may be encountered in daily practice.

The community palliative care clinical nurse specialist may confront attitudes to sickness, life and death that are attributed to the patient's culture. Some cultures view illness as a punishment and believe it is the result of previous wrong doings or committing sinful actions, or perhaps from an evil curse. Other cultures may believe that the patient is possessed by powerful spirits and only an exorcism will cleanse them of the demons. Respect and considerable understanding are required when caring for patients from a different culture to avoid causing alarm or offence. In general, gestures, physical contact, diet, dress, modesty and the expression of both physical and emotional symptoms, as well as customs and ceremonies, can all differ from culture to culture (Brennan 2004). Cultural diversity is not a threatening phenomenon, but it can be challenging for the health care professionals and may bring complexity to the care provided. For all health care professionals, the care of dying patients is one of the most difficult aspects of a clinician's role; however, enabling an individual to die with dignity and providing culturally competent care can be very rewarding (Sheikh and Gatrad 2000).

The most commonly encountered religions within the United Kingdom are Christianity, Judaism, Islam, Hinduism, Sikhism and Buddhism. However, this is by no means a comprehensive list and the community palliative care clinical nurse specialist will not only require a basic knowledge of the above in respect to death and dying, but also need to be prepared to access information on any others encountered within her practice. Within each religion there are also many denominational or sectarian differences and therefore infinite individual variations. It is not necessary for every health care professional caring for a patient to have an in-depth knowledge of each religion and its variations, but to have available further resources for reference should the need arise. What is important is that each patient and family should feel confident and comfortable with the approach of the health care professionals and that any cultural or religious practices and beliefs be respected.

For those dying patients with no religious beliefs, spiritual care is still of paramount importance. Many patients strive to find a sense of peace during the final weeks and days of their life and may require time and encouragement to reflect on their past life. The community palliative care clinical nurse specialist can offer time and listening skills to allow the dying patient to verbalise spiritual issues which may have been previously difficult to express. Enabling patients to communicate their needs and emotions as they move towards the final weeks and days of life can be problematic. Problems may occur due to the nature of the illness, for example neurological damage can make talking difficult and cause distress (Katz and Sidell 1994). Patients suffering from extreme fatigue may find the effort of talking too much of a struggle and some patients will lack confidence or feel embarrassed trying to express themselves. Many individuals will also want to be able to communicate with their family and friends before death approaches. They may want to say final goodbyes and express their love and gratitude to their family. It is therefore important for patients to be informed when death is approaching, to allow them time to complete unfinished business.

The community palliative care clinical nurse specialist can assist patients to communicate by demonstrating a non-judgemental and empathetic approach, encouraging patients through active listening and giving them time to relate their feelings and wishes. The aim will be to allow patients to maintain some degree of autonomy, even when their mental faculties may be declining or as death approaches (Katz and Sidell 1994). The role of health care professionals is to assist dying patients, not only with their physical care, but also incorporating the psychological, cultural and spiritual aspects of dying into the care they provide and helping the patient through this final life transition (Young and Koopsen 2005).

Key Points

- Being at home allows patients a greater opportunity to determine their own care and receiving information about end of life care, discussing complex emotions and communicating with the family are all sensitive issues which the community palliative care clinical nurse specialist can address with the patient.
- No individual can meet all the needs of the patient approaching death and therefore multidisciplinary teamwork lies at the heart of effective palliative care in the home, where the community palliative care clinical nurse specialist works alongside the other members of the primary health care team to deliver a service tailored to the wishes of the dying patient.
- The role of the community palliative care clinical nurse specialist is to assist the district nurse and other members of the primary health care team with complex problems and together ensure that the patient is comfortable and confident to remain in his or her own home until death.
- Many patients will present with complex circumstances and distressing symptoms; these difficult situations are challenging to all the health professionals involved, but effective end of life care can be delivered through anticipating problems, minimising crisis and working together to support patients in their last weeks or days of life.
- As the disease progresses and death approaches, the needs and wishes of the patient may change and it is necessary to continually reassess the situation with the individual to ensure his or her continuing needs are being met.
- For patients facing death, having autonomy and retaining some control over their situation is increasingly important, particularly as they deal with losses in their physical function.
- Religious practices and rituals are of considerable importance when patients wish to remain at home for the final days of their life.
- The community palliative care clinical nurse specialist can assist patients at this difficult time by demonstrating a non-judgemental and empathetic approach, encouraging patients through active listening and giving them time to relate their feelings and wishes.

Useful resources

Dimond B (2004) Disposal and preparation of the body: different religious practices. *British Journal Of Nursing* 13 (9), 547–550.

Kearney N, Richardson A (eds) (2006) *Nursing Patients with Cancer: Principles and Practice.* Elsevier Churchill Livingstone, Edinburgh.

Neuberger J (2004) *Dying Well: A Guide to Enabling a Good Death,* 2nd edn. Radcliffe, Abingdon.

Palmer E, Howarth J (2005) *Palliative Care for the Primary Care Team.* Quay Books, London.

Payne S, Seymour J, Ingleton C (eds) (2004) *Palliative Care Nursing: Principles and Evidence for Practice.* Open University Press, Maidenhead.

Thomas K (2003) *Caring for the Dying at Home: Companions on the Journey.* Radcliffe Medical Press, Abingdon.

References

Barraclough J (1999) *Cancer and Emotion: A Practical Guide to Psycho-Oncology,* 3rd edn. John Wiley and Sons, Chichester.

Booth R (2000) Spirituality: sharing the journey. In: Cooper J (ed) *Stepping into Palliative Care: A Handbook for Community Professionals,* pp 126–135. Radcliffe Medical Press, Abingdon.

Brennan J (2004) *Cancer in Context: A Practical Guide to Supportive Care.* Oxford University Press, Oxford.

Bycroft L, Brown JG (1996) Care of the dying. In: Tschudin V (ed) *Nursing the Patient with Cancer,* 2nd edn, pp 419–437. Prentice Hall International, Hemel Hempstead.

Corr CA, Nabe CM, Corr DM (2003) *Death and Dying: Life and Living,* 4th edn. Thomson Wadsworth, Belmont.

Dimond B (2004) Disposal and preparation of the body: different religious practices. *British Journal of Nursing* 13 (9), 547–550.

Doyle D, Jeffrey D (2000) *Palliative Care in the Home.* Oxford University Press, Oxford.

Dunne K, Sullivan K, Kernohan G (2005) Palliative care for patients with cancer: district nurses' experiences. *Journal of Advanced Nursing* 50 (4), 372–380.

Fisher M (2002) Emotional pain and eliciting concerns. In: Penson J, Fisher RA (eds) *Palliative Care for People with Cancer,* 3rd edn, pp 171–189. Arnold, London.

Furlong E, O'Toole S (2006) Psychological care for patients with cancer. In: Kearney N, Richardson A (eds) *Nursing Patients with Cancer: Principles and Practice,* pp 717–737. Elsevier Churchill Livingstone, Edinburgh.

Henderson M (2004) Anxiety. In: Sykes N, Edmonds P, Wiles J (eds) *Management of Advanced Disease,* 4th edn, pp 65–72. Arnold, London.

Jeffrey D (1998) Communication skills in palliative care. In: Faull C, Carter Y, Woof R (eds) *Handbook of Palliative Care*, pp 88–98. Blackwell Science, Oxford.

Jeffrey D (2000) *Cancer: From Cure to Care. Palliative Care Dilemmas in General Practice*. Hochland and Hochland, Manchester.

Jeffrey D (2003) What do we mean by psychosocial care in palliative care. In: Lloyd-Williams M (ed) *Psychosocial Issues in Palliative Care*, pp 1–12. Oxford University Press, Oxford.

Johnston G (2004) Social death: the impact of protracted dying. In: Payne S, Seymour J, Ingleton C (eds) *Palliative Care Nursing: Principles and Evidence for Practice*, pp 351–363. Open University Press, Maidenhead.

Katz J, Sidell M (1994) *Easeful Death: Caring for Dying and Bereaved People*. Hodder and Stoughton, London.

Kemp C (1999) *Terminal Illness: A Guide to Nursing Care*, 2nd edn. Lippincott, Philadelphia.

Kibler S (1996) Counselling. In: Tschudin V (ed) *Nursing the Patient with Cancer*, 2nd edn, pp 452–467. Prentice Hall, Hemel Hempstead.

Lakasing E, Mahaffey W (2006) Caring for the dying patient at home. *Geriatric Medicine* 36 (3), 21–22, 25–26, 28.

Lee E (2002) *In Your Own Time: A Guide for Patients and Their Carers Facing a Last Illness at Home*. Oxford University Press, Oxford.

Lloyd-Williams M (ed) (2003) *Psychosocial Issues in Palliative Care*. Oxford University Press, Oxford.

McIntyre R, Lugton J (2005) Supporting the family and carers. In: Lugton J, McIntyre R (eds) *Palliative Care: The Nursing Role*, 2nd edn, pp 261–301. Elsevier Churchill Livingstone, Edinburgh.

Mirando S (2006) Palliative care. In: Kearney N, Richardson A (eds) *Nursing Patients with Cancer: Principles and Practice*, pp 821–848. Elsevier Churchill Livingstone. Edinburgh.

Neuberger J (2004) *Dying Well: A Guide to Enabling a Good Death*, 2nd edn. Radcliffe, Abingdon.

Palmer E, Howarth J (2005) *Palliative Care for the Primary Care Team*. Quay Books, London.

Payne S, Seymour J, Ingleton C (2004) Introduction. In: Payne S. Seymour J, Ingleton C (eds) *Palliative Care Nursing: Principles and Evidence for Practice*, pp 1–12. Open University Press, Maidenhead.

Proot IM, Abu-Saad HH, Meulen RHJ, Goldsteen M, Spreeuwenberg C, Widdershoven GAM (2004) The needs of terminally ill patients at home: directing one's life, health and things related to beloved others. *Palliative Medicine* 18 (1), 53–61.

Regnard C, Tempest S (1998) *A Guide to Symptom Relief in Advanced Disease*. Hochland and Hochland, Hale.

Royal College of Nursing (2002) *A Framework for Nurses Working in Specialist Palliative Care*. Competencies Project, Royal College of Nursing, London.

Sahlberg-Blom E, Ternestedt BM, Johansson JE (1998) The last month of life: continuity, care site and place of death. *Palliative Medicine* 12 (4), 287–296.

Sheikh A, Gatrad AR (2000) Death and bereavement: an exploration and a meditation. In: Sheikh A, Gatrad AR (eds) *Caring for Muslim Patients*, pp 97–109. Radcliffe Medical Press, Abingdon.

Sheldon F (1997) *Psychosocial Palliative Care: Good Practice in the Care of the Dying and Bereaved*. Stanley Thornes, Cheltenham.

Sheldon F (2004) Communication. In: Sykes N, Edmonds P, Wiles J (eds) *Management of Advanced Disease*, 4th edn, pp 9–26. Arnold, London.

Thomas K (2003) *Caring for the Dying at Home: Companions on the Journey*. Radcliffe Medical Press, Abingdon.

Twycross R (1999) *Introducing Palliative Care*, 3rd edn. Radcliffe Medical Press, Abingdon.

Wells M (2001) The impact of cancer. In: Corner J, Bailey C (eds)*Cancer Nursing: Care in Context*, pp 63–85. Blackwell Science, Oxford.

Wilkie P (1998) The person, the patient and their carers. In: Faull C, Carter Y, Woof R (eds) *Handbook of Palliative Care*, pp 55–63. Blackwell Science, Oxford.

Wong FKY, Liu CF, Szeto Y, Sham M, Chan T (2004) Health problems encountered by dying patients receiving palliative home care until death. *Cancer Nursing* 27 (3), 244–251.

Young C, Koopsen C (2005) *Spirituality, Health and Healing*. Jones and Bartlett, Sudbury.

Dying at Home: Addressing the Practical Needs

Introduction

Dying at home can be problematic; however, many of the difficulties encountered in the last days of life can be predicted and resolved quickly by an effective health care team. The patient's needs are continually assessed and interventions individualised to that patient. Communication is of vital importance to ensure that all members of the team are kept abreast of the situation, including out-of-hours services. Within the home, the patient and family members may worry about the daily practicalities such as drug administration, fluids, nutrition, hygiene needs, incontinence, etc. The practical problems of 'wanting to die at home' are easier to overcome if the patient and family have been well informed in advance and have an awareness of potential difficulties. They require information about the practicalities of providing direct care to the patient and also contact numbers for the various nursing and medical services should assistance be required. The community palliative care clinical nurse specialist has a role in discussing end of life care with patients and answering questions about their concerns and anticipated problems. The objective is to provide patients with adequate information about the care available to allow them to live as autonomously as possible, up until the time of death (Sahlberg-Blom et al. 1998).

Practical aspects of dying at home

Dying at home allows patients to be nursed in familiar surroundings and to have their loved ones care for them physically, as well as offering supportive care. Most individuals have a natural desire to die at home, providing they can be looked after properly, because this is where they feel secure and safe (Reoch1997). However, this process can be fraught with difficulties and many problems may be encountered which had not been previously imagined by patients or their carers. Dying at home may fulfil the patient's need to be with relatives and the death to be a positive experience, but it has to be matched by the family's ability to provide the care over what may be a prolonged period (Costello 2004). The role of the community palliative care clinical nurse specialist may be to discuss end of life care with anxious patients and/or their relatives. Although patients will be informed about the dying process and the associated weakness, few patients can envisage what this means or the loss of independence that ensues. Whilst the focus of discussion may centre on the physical symptoms associated with dying, such as pain, nausea and vomiting, breathlessness, fatigue, etc., it may be difficult to relay to patients, and for patients to understand, the practicalities of requiring assistance with personal hygiene, assistance with toileting, possible continence problems, assistance with feeding or transferring in and out of bed.

Whilst reassurance can be given to patients that services such as the district nursing team and social service carers will be able to provide assistance with many of the aspects of care, they are unable to provide that care 24 hours per day. Patients soon discover that the care required does not always coincide with visits from the professionals and they become ever more reliant on their loved ones for assistance with tasks such as toileting, etc. This can place the burden of care on the family, and result in ever-increasing feelings of loss and helplessness by the patient.

Case Story: Josephine

Josephine lived alone in a private sheltered housing complex. Her daughter had two children and lived about 10 miles away; she visited as often as possible. Josephine had advanced lung cancer and wished to remain at home to die. Initially this was very successful, with visits from social carers and the district nurses daily. The community palliative care clinical nurse specialist had a call from Josephine's daughter to express her concerns that her mother was no longer safe at home after a number of falls whilst going to the toilet. The daughter was getting increasing calls during the day and night to respond to Josephine's alarm system. She felt she was no longer able to give this level of care to her mother and was becoming very tired.

Josephine refused to consider any other place of care and reported to the community palliative care clinical nurse specialist that she would manage. However, after several difficult weeks Josephine began to express feelings of guilt about the burden of care she was placing on her exhausted daughter and felt she could no longer expect her to come day and night in response to her emergency calls. Josephine felt helpless and no longer able to care for herself. She reluctantly agreed to try Marie Curie nurses overnight and found this improved the situation considerably. Josephine no longer felt so dependent and had regained a degree of control. The relationship with her daughter improved and Josephine remained at home until she died a few days later.

The care of patients who want to remain at home can be difficult when family members become exhausted. Not all patients are willing to accept help from the professionals and continue to rely on the family to support them. Careful negotiation and good communication skills are necessary to stop potentially volatile situations from arising. Carers and family members may feel they can no longer cope with the demands of caring and they insist the patient goes to hospital. The community palliative care clinical nurse specialist will use her wealth of experience to allow both the patient, who may be extremely weak and frail, and the family to express their feelings and try to work out a solution that will be acceptable to both parties. This will be intended to allow the patient his or her wish to remain at home and also to relieve the family of some of the caring. Many of the practical tasks of caring for the dying patient at home will be undertaken by family members and this can prove difficult or embarrassing. Patients and their families do not receive palliative care training; they may have no prior knowledge or experience and this may be the first time the relative/family member has had to perform care of an intimate nature on another adult, let alone their own mother or father, etc. The community palliative care clinical nurse specialist will offer time to explore the difficulties the carers may be experiencing and also to discuss strategies that may make the situation more agreeable to the patient and family.

Case Story: Doreen

Doreen was 76 years of age and had always been very independent. Her family lived next door and visited daily. Doreen had advanced metastatic lung cancer. As her condition deteriorated, the family

---

Case Story: Doreen (*continued*)

were aware of her difficulties in performing some of the activities of living, such as personal hygiene and meal preparation. Doreen refused any help and reported being able to care for herself. As the weeks passed, the community palliative care clinical nurse specialist became increasingly concerned for Doreen and eventually persuaded her to take some assistance from the social services. This was mainly for medication prompting and meal assistance. Doreen was a very private individual and adamantly refused to allow her daughter to provide any care, especially assistance with personal hygiene. Doreen expressed her horror and embarrassment at the thought of anyone having to provide assistance with intimate, personal care, especially her own daughter. When Doreen became bed bound, the health care team found it increasingly difficult to provide the level of care required 24 hours a day without the assistance of the family. However, in accordance with Doreen's wishes, her daughter sat at her bedside, but provided no physical care. As weakness took its toll on Doreen, she eventually allowed the district nursing team to assist with all her care needs. Her daughter expressed her frustration at not being allowed to help in her mother's care, but could also understand why her mother found it difficult. Doreen's daughter also confessed to the community palliative care clinical nurse specialist at being a little relieved that her mother did not want her to participate in the care, as she felt she would have been embarrassed herself and that it would have taken away her mother's last remnants of dignity and privacy.

Taking the patient's wishes into consideration can, at times, create problems and difficulties in providing care; the community palliative care clinical nurse specialist has an important part to play in listening to the patient and allowing the patient's voice to be heard. The practical aspects of care should always be aimed at allowing patients to maintain some independence and participation in their care. A variety of professionals may be able to offer assistance to try to promote the patient's independence, even if only for a short time. Help may be elicited from the physiotherapist to assess for walking aids and this may allow patients to maintain their mobility for just a few weeks or days longer and allow them the privacy of the bathroom for toileting. The occupational therapist may assist with the provision of bathing aids, such as an hydraulic bath seat, to allow patients the luxury of easing their aches and pains in the warm water and again providing some independence and a sense of achievement. Many other pieces of equipment may be provided, from a variety of sources, all aimed at maintaining patient safety and comfort. These may include a commode, raised toilet seat, pressure-relieving mattress and cushion, hoist, grab rails and chair raisers. Difficulties sometimes arise, however, when family members feel they may have lost control of their own home as it slowly starts to resemble a hospital, with bits of equipment everywhere. It is important that the health care professionals supply only what is necessary and, as the patient's condition deteriorates, remove any pieces that are no longer of use.

Case Story: George

George was now in the final days of his life. He was being cared for at home by his wife and the district nursing team. He was comfortable and enjoying the company of his wife at his bedside. However, his wife and their two sons were finding all the equipment in the house a constant reminder of George's weakening condition and wanted it all taken away. There were rails, a bath seat, a perching stool and a toilet raiser in the bathroom; a commode in the landing cupboard; a Zimmer frame at the top of the stairs; seat raisers in the lounge, on George's favourite chair; and a perching stool in the kitchen. One of the sons became particularly angry each time he saw equipment that his father would no longer be able to use. A special request was made to the equipment loan store to come that day and uplift as much as possible. The family were grateful when it was no longer in the house and felt they could now concentrate their attention on George, rather than getting upset and angry at the equipment and the losses that it represented.

Feelings of isolation and loss

Patients choosing to die at home may also face difficulties with isolation and feeling *distanced* from their family. As patients become progressively weaker, tasks such as walking become more difficult and they become gradually housebound. This can bring a sense of loss and a feeling of being very alone. This may be further exaggerated as their weakness progresses and they spend more time in bed. The bedroom may be upstairs or away from the main living areas within the house and the patient no longer feels part of the family. Sensitive discussion with the patient and family may allow for the bed to be brought into the living room, enabling the dying patient to remain part of family life (Langford 1995). However, this may also result in a loss of privacy for both the patient and family members. Toileting, personal hygiene needs, etc. may become embarrassing with a loss of modesty and dignity, whilst the family no longer have *space* to conduct their own lives. Careful planning and discussion between the patient, family and community palliative care clinical nurse specialist prior to the patient's deterioration may have partly prepared everyone for these eventualities.

The physical losses that dying patients have to endure may be overwhelming and result in patients feeling helpless and *useless*. They may not be able to walk about freely and must rely on others for help; they may lose physical strength which makes even simple tasks difficult or impossible; the inability to perform personal intimate care may result in a loss of privacy and modesty; they may also have difficulties with bowel or bladder function, which, for many patients, is embarrassing and undignified. These practical losses may also be accompanied by physical symptoms which will compound the patient's difficulties. The common symptoms associated with dying are weakness, anorexia, nausea and vomiting, constipation, breathlessness and pain. The role of the community palliative care clinical specialist, in conjunction with the primary health care team, is to maximise symptom control and alleviate the patient's distress where possible. Good symptom management, in many instances, will promote a sense of well-being and allow the dying patient to regain some physical function.

Case Story: Jimmy

Jimmy was only 58 years of age and was very angry with life. He had been a successful businessman and had just retired. He had made many plans with his wife, about their future together and all the long holidays they were going to have. He was now dying from metastatic prostate cancer. Not only did he have physical symptoms from pain, constipation and overwhelming fatigue, but also he found the role of dying patient hard to accept. He felt embarrassed and helpless, unable to even go to the toilet alone. His psychological and spiritual distress were being expressed by anger and he refused to see anyone other than immediate family. His wife found his anger difficult to accept and would have liked more support, but respected Jimmy's wishes that no-one else see him in this sad state. The community palliative care clinical nurse specialist was asked by the general practitioner to visit Jimmy and assess the whole situation. Jimmy was reluctant to vocalise his feelings or indeed his symptoms; he perceived expressing pain as a weakness. On the second visit to Jimmy he suddenly broke down and sobbed uncontrollably. This allowed both himself and his wife to express the emotions that had been suppressed for many weeks. Jimmy reported that pain was at times unbearable and he found the whole situation embarrassing and undignified. With Jimmy's consent, Marie Curie nurses were organised to give his wife a break, social carers were enlisted to help with personal care and the district nurses increased their visits. His constipation was alleviated and the severe pain addressed with a change in analgesia. Jimmy agreed to see some of his friends and this relieved his feelings of isolation from the outside world. He managed to regain some mobility when his pain was better controlled and for a short time could toilet himself. The situation had improved for both Jimmy and his wife; he even managed to plan his funeral, regaining some control of what was happening. Having gained relief from his pain, improved symptom control and had an opportunity to express and discuss his emotions, Jimmy was able to die peacefully at home.

Finalising affairs

Dying patients will require not only assistance with their physical care, but also an opportunity to organise their affairs and discuss their approaching death. Many individuals will want to broach topics that may be difficult to discuss with their loved ones, for example their funeral, future care needs of the family or indeed who is going to support an elderly spouse or young children. The community palliative care clinical nurse specialist may have to act as facilitator to allow the patient to discuss these emotional issues with the family. This has to be undertaken before the patient becomes too weak and finds it impossible to concentrate on the topics; therefore it is essential that the health care professionals are open and honest with the patient when it is evident that death is not far away. Many dying patients find comfort in organising their funeral. This not only allows them some control of what will happen, but also ensures that their wishes will be honoured. Dying patients may want to see a solicitor, to organise a will or put their affairs in order. If the patient lives alone and has no family in attendance, it may be necessary for the community palliative care clinical nurse specialist to contact the undertaker or solicitor and arrange for them to visit the patient.

Case Story: Judy

Judy was a single parent. Her son had just reached his 18th birthday and was due to go to university soon. Judy's parents were elderly and had their own health problems. Judy had advanced pancreatic cancer and was now in her last days of life. She asked the community palliative care clinical nurse specialist if it would be appropriate to speak to an undertaker. Together they agreed it would and the community palliative care clinical nurse specialist contacted the local funeral directors and asked them to visit at a time when Judy would be alone in the house. Judy did not want to upset her son or parents if they saw the undertaker in the house prior to her death. She had very fixed views on her funeral and appreciated being given the opportunity to arrange things the way she wanted. After Judy died, her son and parents were greatly relieved to discover that Judy had made the arrangements, as they had always found it too painful to even try to approach the subject.

The age and stage of life an individual has reached may determine the practical issues related to death. The elderly may have consulted a solicitor many years before their illness developed, or indeed planned and paid for their funeral. Younger patients may not have envisaged the need for such arrangements as they had assumed life would stretch out before them for many years. Contemplating and organising their own funeral, ensuring their affairs are in order or making arrangements for their children then becomes a very traumatic and painful experience for the individuals. Good supportive care is necessary to assist the dying patient at this time, and the community palliative care clinical nurse specialist may be the professional that the individual selects to assist in this process. Dying patients and those caring for them have special needs and these can best be met by professionals with special expertise (Corr et al. 2003).

The final days

Dying patients who are entering the final phase of their illness have health needs that require particular expertise. The general practitioner and district nurse will be heavily involved in the care and support of the patient at this time, with the community palliative care clinical nurse specialist providing direct or indirect care to the patient. The involvement of the community palliative care clinical nurse specialist is intended to complement the care provided by the other members of the primary health care team and may consist of advice, information or support to colleagues, as well as direct care to the patient and family. A team approach is necessary, with good communication between the professionals and regular review of the patient's symptoms being paramount. The patient's condition may change rapidly as death approaches and therefore the intervention requires to be responsive and adaptable. A tool such as the Liverpool Care Pathway (Ellershaw and Wilkinson 2003) may be of great benefit to all the health professionals involved in caring for the patient in the final days of life. Anticipating needs, actively preventing problems and successful care planning is the key to effective care of the dying patient.

Recognising the last days of a patient's life is not always easy, even for experienced health care professionals. However, common to most patients is a gradual weakening of their body, feeling increasingly tired, increased periods of sleep, gradual loss of function and their voice may become little more than a whisper. They will have little interest in food or fluids, may have continence problems and will require assistance with all aspects of care. Their appearance may alter due to weight loss, their skin may take on a faded or pale appearance, the face may look gaunt and the extremities may be cooler to the touch (Atkinson and Virdee 2001). The individual may also become disorientated to time and place, may have difficulty concentrating and at times may become agitated and confused. Regular information and explanations should be given to the patient and family to increase their understanding at this time and also to allow the family to be as involved in the patient's care as they wish to be. Caring for a loved one through the last days of life can be a great gift or terrible burden (Palmer and Howarth 2005); it is therefore incumbent on the health care professionals to ensure the carer and family have all the resources available to maintain the patient at home.

Case Story: David

David was in the last few days of his life. His wife and family were now exhausted as he had been unwell for 3 years and for the past 4 months had required a lot of assistance. He wished to remain at home, but was not sleeping well at night and could not bear to be

---

Case Story: David (*continued*)

alone. This was placing considerable strain on a very tired family. The community palliative care clinical nurse specialist discussed the problems with his wife and himself. He was now very weak and evidently dying. He asked not to be moved anywhere, he desperately wanted to die at home. He agreed to allow Marie Curie nurses to sit with him at night to allow his wife and family some respite. He was reassured his wife was only in the next room and would come if needed. He was also happy for the district nurses to provide his personal care, again relieving his wife of that duty. With the increased services, his wife was able to take a break, but still be around if needed. David died 2 days later at home, in the company of his wife and family.

The aim of care in the final days of life is to allow the patient to die with dignity, to be comfortable and in the place of his or her choosing. It is therefore essential for the health care professionals to regularly review the care and also to ensure the family are being given adequate support in their caring role. Support and companionship to the patient and family are essential at this time. Symptom control is of paramount importance and the community palliative care clinical nurse specialist will be able to give expert advice on a variety of symptoms. Many patients by this stage in their illness will have difficulty with or be unable to take oral medication and it may be necessary to use a syringe driver to achieve relief of their symptoms such as pain, nausea or agitation. It is also good practice to discontinue drugs that no longer benefit the dying patient and administer only essential medication. The role of the community palliative care clinical nurse specialist is to ensure that both the patient and family have been prepared for this stage in the illness and discussions will have taken place previously about medication and the use of the syringe driver. Many patients and their families negatively associate the use of the syringe driver with approaching death, but careful explanation about its use, at an earlier stage in the illness, will avert any fears or concerns. It will also allow patients to remain at home who may otherwise have had to go into hospital or a hospice for symptom control.

Cultural and religious issues

As discussed in the previous chapter, consideration has to be given to the various cultural and religious practices that the health care team may encounter whilst caring for dying patients at home. Considerable care has to be taken to avoid causing offence or embarrassment to the patient. For example, some Asians consider it disrespectful to look someone in the eye and may avoid direct eye contact with the health care professionals, whilst Middle Eastern countries perceive eye contact between a man and woman as having sexual connotations (Brennan 2004). Modesty is also of great importance, particularly for women from Arab cultures, where to bare any part of the body, even an arm, would be unthinkable if a male was present (Sheldon 1997). The community palliative care clinical nurse specialist may be required to inform and educate other health care professionals and social services personnel of the customs and practices of such patients to ensure culturally sensitive care, particularly in relation to personal hygiene needs.

Food is another source of cultural difference. The dietary needs of the dying patient may be limited, but again consideration needs to be given to any special dietary requirements or the preparation of such foods in accordance with the patient's cultural or religious beliefs, particularly if the patient lives alone and social services are assisting with meal preparation. The prescribing of nutritional sip feeds may be inappropriate for some patients where their religion or culture makes it difficult to modify their diet. Periods of religious fasting may also impinge on the administration of drugs to the dying patient.

For many individuals, religious belief has special meaning as they approach death (Booth 2000). The health care professionals need to take care not to breach any of the religious tenets and will appreciate guidance and support from the patient's family or faith leader. Patients of the Christian faith may wish to see a chaplain or priest to have Holy Communion or anointing of the sick performed. A rabbi will visit Jewish patients and hear the deathbed confession and repentance (Kemp 1999). Jewish families will remain at the bedside to support the patient during the final days and will want to be present at the moment of death.

The presence of a Hindu priest is comforting to followers of the Hindu faith and rituals include prayers and chanting. Relatives will welcome an opportunity to sit with the dying patient and read from a Holy book. Modesty is of great importance to Hindus and may extend to women refusing care unless their husband is present. The patient may also wish to die on the floor near Mother Earth. Death at home is preferable for the Hindu and the eldest son will be expected to be present.

Buddhists may find comfort from a priest or monk who may chant and burn incense at a patient's bedside. The Buddhist also wishes to retain mental clarity and may refuse analgesics which induce drowsiness. Sikhs will appreciate privacy for personal prayers and as death approaches Sikh scriptures are read (Twycross 1999). The five symbols of the faith should also be respected: the uncut hair, comb and turban, metal bangle, special knee-length underwear and their dagger (often worn as a brooch).

The dying Muslim usually wants to be nursed at home and will be visited by family and friends who pray for the patient's welfare in the life to come; close family will remain at the bedside reciting from the Qur'an (Sheikh and Gatrad 2000). Cleanliness is of great importance to Muslims, who believe in washing their mouths, hands and feet five times daily before prayers; bed-bound patients may need assistance in this respect, however health care professionals should be aware that personal hygiene provided by individuals of a different gender may be distressing to Muslims (Kemp 1999). Muslim patients also prefer to lie facing Mecca and the room should be rearranged to accommodate their wishes.

District nursing staff in particular, because of their practical nursing role, may find it helpful to discuss issues with the patient and family prior to the final weeks or days of life and therefore be more familiar with any cultural or religious practices and rituals. The role of the community palliative care clinical nurse specialist may be as a resource for other health professionals, but also to offer the patient and family an opportunity to express their needs, discuss pertinent concerns, such as Buddhists and their beliefs regarding mental clarity and analgesia, give reassurance and relay the patient's wishes to the other health care team members.

Case Story: Gertrude

Gertrude was 84 years of age and now in the last weeks of life from a metastatic breast cancer. She lived alone, but had a very caring son who visited as often as possible. She belonged to a religious group that believed in the power of prayer and having a positive attitude to illness and ill health. Her son wanted reassurance that his mother's religious convictions would be taken into consideration as her condition deteriorated. She would accept simple pain relief only (paracetamol), believing that her pain was a state of mind. The community palliative care clinical nurse specialist discussed with Gertrude her wishes and relayed these to the other members of the team. It was only in the last 2 days of her life that she agreed to a small amount of opiate analgesia. She died very peacefully with her son by her bedside.

The health care team and, in particular, district nursing staff may also be present at or around the time of a patient's death at home. Important rituals and religious practices also surround the death and preparation of the body for burial or cremation. Again these will be in accordance with the patient's faith. It is essential that health care professionals, in particular any nursing staff present at the time of death, recognise the importance for the patient and family of the rituals and comply with requests from the family.

After a Jewish person dies, a member of the Jewish community will usually wash the body, the eyes are closed, the body is laid on the floor and candles are lit around the body; the deceased is never left alone until after the burial (Dimond 2004). It is advisable for any health professional to wear gloves to avoid direct contact with the body (Twycross 1999). Following the death of a Muslim, the body must not be touched by a non-Muslim (Kemp 1999). A family member of the same gender or designated Muslim from the community will wash the body. Muslims view death as part of a journey to meet their God (Young and Koopsen 2005); the funeral takes place very quickly and may be within a few hours of the death. The body of a Sikh is washed and dressed by family members following death; however, there is no objection to health professionals handling the body. The body of a Hindu will be placed so that the head is facing south, incense burned and religious pictures turned to the wall and in some traditions mirrors are also covered (Dimond 2004). The body is usually washed by family members and dressed in new clothes. There are no specific rituals relating to the washing and preparation of Buddhists after death, although in many instances the family will attend to the body.

All of these religious rituals are of considerable significance to the families of the deceased, and although they may be unfamiliar to some or all of the health professionals involved in the patient's care, they are important aspects of care and will ultimately help the family in their grief knowing that the patient's wishes have been respected and rituals carried out in accordance with their faith.

Therefore, not only is it important to address the physical symptoms that may be associated with dying, but also spiritual and psychological issues may still be of concern to the patient. Communication may become more difficult and, as the voice weakens, it may not always be possible to understand what the patient is saying. However, the patient may appreciate the company of the health care professional just sitting by the bedside and showing care and understanding at this difficult time. This is a time for allowing individuals and their loved ones time and privacy to say final goodbyes; thus nursing and medical intervention should be kept to a minimum. Family members may be frightened and tired, but most will appreciate the opportunity to express their emotions. The community palliative care clinical nurse specialist can take time to sit with the family and allow them the opportunity to discuss their fears. However, the visits from the health care professionals should be discussed and co-ordinated to cause the least disruption to the family at this *special* time.

Dying at home presents challenges for patients, their families and the professionals involved in the individual's care. There is a need for support and excellent nursing and medical care to give the patient a *good* death. The community palliative care clinical nurse specialist can offer intervention to all parties, both directly and indirectly, making the transition from life to death, caring to grieving, as smooth as possible.

Key Points

- Many of the practical tasks of caring for the dying patient at home will be undertaken by family members and this can prove difficult or embarrassing.
- Dying patients will require not only assistance with their physical care, but also an opportunity to organise their affairs and discuss their approaching death.
- The patient's condition may change rapidly as death approaches and therefore the intervention requires to be responsive and adaptable.
- The aim of care in the final days of life is to allow patients to die with dignity, to be comfortable and in the place of their choosing.
- The community palliative care clinical nurse specialist can offer intervention to all parties, both directly and indirectly, making the transition from life to death, caring to grieving, as smooth as possible.

Useful resources

Dimond B (2004) Disposal and preparation of the body: different religious practices. *British Journal of Nursing* 13 (9), 547–550.

Ellershaw JE, Wilkinson S (2003) *Care of the Dying: A Pathway to Excellence.* Oxford University Press, Oxford.

Kearney N, Richardson A (eds) (2006) *Nursing Patients with Cancer: Principles and Practice.* Elsevier Churchill Livingstone, Edinburgh.

Neuberger J (2004) *Dying Well: A Guide to Enabling a Good Death*, 2nd edn. Radcliffe, Abingdon.

Palmer E, Howarth J (2005) *Palliative Care for the Primary Care Team*. Quay Books, London.

Payne S, Seymour J, Ingleton C (eds) (2004) *Palliative Care Nursing: Principles and Evidence for Practice*. Open University Press, Maidenhead.

Thomas K (2003) *Caring for the Dying at Home: Companions on the Journey*. Radcliffe Medical Press, Abingdon.

References

Atkinson J, Virdee A (2001) Promoting comfort for patients with symptoms other than pain. In: Kinghorn S, Gamlin R (eds) *Palliative Nursing: Bringing Comfort and Hope*, pp 43–62. Bailliere Tindall, London.

Booth R (2000) Spirituality: sharing the journey. In: Cooper J (ed) *Stepping into Palliative Care: A Handbook for Community Professionals*, pp 126–135. Radcliffe Medical Press, Abingdon.

Brennan J (2004) *Cancer in Context: A Practical Guide to Supportive Care*. Oxford University Press, Oxford.

Corr CA, Nabe CM, Corr DM (2003) *Death and Dying: Life and Living*, 4th edn. Thomson Wadsworth, Belmont.

Costello J (2004) *Nursing the Dying Patient: Caring in Different Contexts*. Palgrave Macmillan, Basingstoke.

Dimond B (2004) Disposal and preparation of the body: different religious practices. *British Journal of Nursing* 13 (9), 547–550.

Doyle D, Jeffrey D (2000) *Palliative Care in the Home*. Oxford University Press, Oxford.

Ellershaw JE, Wilkinson S (2003) *Care of the Dying: A Pathway to Excellence*. Oxford University Press, Oxford.

Kemp C (1999) *Terminal Illness: A Guide to Nursing Care*, 2nd edn. Lippincott, Philadelphia.

Langford L (1995) Care in the home. In: Robbins J, Moscrop J (eds) *Caring for the Dying Patient and the Family*, 3rd edn, pp 208–222. Chapman and Hall, London.

Palmer E, Howarth J (2005) *Palliative Care for the Primary Care Team*. Quay Books, London.

Reoch R (1997) *Dying Well: A Holistic Guide for the Dying and Their Carers*. Gaia, London.

Sahlberg-Blom E, Ternestedt BM, Johansson JE (1998) The last month of life: continuity, care site and place of death. *Palliative Medicine* 12 (4), 287–296.

Sheikh A, Gatrad AR (2000) Death and bereavement: an exploration and a meditation. In: Sheikh A, Gatrad AR (eds) *Caring for Muslim Patients*, pp 97–109. Radcliffe Medical Press, Abingdon.

Sheldon F (1997) *Psychosocial Palliative Care: Good Practice in the Care of the Dying and Bereaved*. Stanley Thornes, Cheltenham.

Twycross R (1999) *Introducing Palliative Care*, 3rd edn. Radcliffe Medical Press, Abingdon.

Young C, Koopsen C (2005) *Spirituality, Health and Healing*. Jones and Bartlett, Sudbury.

Section III
Carers

What Do Carers Do? **7**

Introduction

As a result of demographic changes, care in the community for those with a chronic or life-threatening illness is now required on a scale not previously imagined. Chronic means an illness for which a cure is not currently available (Payne and Ellis-Hill 2001) and therefore the individual will be unable to return to his or her former way of life. This growing number of individuals living at home with an ongoing illness has resulted in the family now being the primary resource for looking after the chronically ill. This has major economic implications for the UK government.

According to Payne and Ellis-Hill (2001), the range of roles covered by informal carers can vary from monitoring a person's environment to ensure their safety, to 24 hours a day hands-on personal care of a highly dependent individual. This will vary from person to person depending on the stage of the patient's illness, but as in any chronic illness the trajectory of dying is unclear and carers face the emotional uncertainty of the weeks and months ahead.

Palliative care also presents additional complexity where physical decline may be rapid, giving the carer little time to adapt to the escalating demands of the caring role and the impending death of the patient (Zapart et al. 2007). The needs of the carer and family have to be taken into consideration with regards to their quality of life, as the caring role has implications for their employment, finances, family life and social contacts. Palliative care encompasses the needs of the family as well as the patient and therefore specialist psychosocial support can also be given to the carer by the community palliative care clinical nurse specialist.

The role of the carer

Family members and informal carers are the single most important resource for looking after patients at home with a long-term or life-threatening illness. This also extends to those patients with end-stage disease who have a shorter illness trajectory, but have chosen to remain at home for the duration of their illness and, more importantly, to die at home. Today, it is members of the family who are increasingly replacing skilled health care professionals in the delivery of unfamiliar, complex care (Aoun et al. 2005). When an individual is diagnosed with a life-threatening illness, the impact is immediately felt within the family and they are required to adapt their daily lives to support the patient. Many studies have shown that today's carers are seen to be carrying a heavy burden with considerable costs to themselves in terms of health, well-being and financial security (Coote 1996; Altschuler et al. 1997; Lubkin and Payne 1998; Edwards and Scheetz 2002).

Carers are usually family members, they are unpaid, untrained and provide the care as a consequence of their pre-existing relationship with the patient (Smith 2001). Many carers are isolated and lack support, have financial difficulties and are unable to continue with their paid employment. Most carers perform their caregiving role out of a sense of love or responsibility to the patient (Greenberg et al. 1992); however, many of them have little option because there is no realistic alternative. Unfortunately, health and social services cannot meet the needs of 24-hour care in the home for every patient and patients rely heavily on families to fill in the gaps. Indeed, if families were unable to meet the demands of caring, then the health and social services would face certain crisis. There is no guarantee, however, that in the future the family will be there to perform the caring role. Because of the changes in socio-demographics, with increasing numbers of the very old, changes in family patterns, increasing female employment and geographical mobility, assumptions can no longer be made that family members will be readily available to care for the patient (Payne and Ellis-Hill 2001).

Today's carers include school-age children managing household chores and personal tasks; mothers looking after an elderly parent; male carers who may have to provide ongoing personal care to a spouse or parent; as well as elderly partners facing caregiving demands and their own ageing process (Edwards and Scheetz 2002). At times, caregivers may need more support than the patient and adequate attention should be paid to their physical and emotional needs. Symptoms of depression, anxiety, feelings of helplessness, lowered morale and emotional exhaustion are all associated with caregiving (Greenberg et al. 1992).

Health care professionals need to be aware of the impact on the carer and ensure assistance is on offer in terms of practical help and respite, but also emotionally to prevent the onset of possible mental health problems.

Demands of caring

The majority of families will want to take care of their own loved ones and usually the care given in the home is indeed by a close relative. However, this may prove difficult for the family if they are attempting to balance the demands of the illness and family life. The carer and family will experience numerous losses as a result of their loved one's diagnosis and these may include loss of future plans, loss of being an *ordinary* family and a loss of freedom. Middle-aged women can be particularly affected as they may have children to look after, an ongoing responsibility towards elderly parents, paid employment to maintain and the patient's care needs to be fulfilled (Eriksson and Svedlund 2006).

Case Story: Sophie

Sophie's sister lived alone and was dying from metastatic breast cancer. Sophie had three young children and a husband who worked away from home 2–3 days a week. Sophie's parents were still alive and lived nearby, but her mother suffered a stroke several years ago and her father cared for her mother. Sophie was always very involved in supporting her parents, but now was required to help her sister in her last few weeks of life. She was always seen as being able to cope with the demands of life; however, she was now trying to maintain her own household, care for her children and look after her parents and sister. Sophie's sister mentioned to the general practitioner that she thought Sophie was struggling with all the demands being placed upon her; she had been short tempered with her father and appeared forgetful and exhausted to her sister. Sophie's sister asked if the community palliative care clinical nurse specialist could visit when she knew Sophie would be there, as she felt that Sophie needed support. When the community palliative care clinical nurse specialist visited, Sophie broke down and reported feeling completely overwhelmed by the whole situation. Strategies had to be worked out to ease the

---

Case Story: Sophie (*continued*)

burden. It was agreed, with her parent's permission, to organise social services to help care for her mother and father for a few weeks; the district nursing team also provided extra nursing help for her sister and the social worker was able to initiate help with Sophie's children after school. This allowed Sophie quality time with her sister and relieved her of the worry of her parents.

This scenario illustrates the importance of liaison between the community palliative care clinical nurse specialist and the other members of the wider care team. It is essential for the community palliative care clinical nurse specialist to have a good knowledge of the local health and social services and to facilitate communication and collaborative working; to not only enhance the care of the dying patient, but also offer support in both practical and emotional terms to the carer with complex needs.

Many carers assume that they should be able to face the burden of caregiving competently on their own; however, advances in medical skills and expertise have resulted in patients living with previously untreatable illnesses not only for months, but in some instances for years. Improvements in cancer treatment, for example, have resulted in some patients living with the diagnosis for many years and there is evidence that families are heavily involved in the process of living with the cancer. This can place considerable strain on the family. Sources of stress may include uncertainty about treatments, an absence of knowledge about the caring role, perceived difficulties regarding medication administration and nursing care, and a lack of knowledge about death and dying.

Altschuler et al. (1997) identified that patients are released from hospitals far more ill and disabled than previously, so that caring for a family member at home may require complex skills and be a considerable challenge. Consequently, it may be necessary to pose the question regarding the extent to which carers are offered real choices about their level of involvement in caring for the patient and what ability do they have to refuse if the personal and family costs seem simply too high? Many families agree to look after their loved one at home because that is what the patient has requested; however, the family may have little insight into the caring role and the significant implications for the whole family. Many families take on the caring role either by default, because no-one else is available to give the care, or in a crisis situation, when they just have to get on with it (Payne and Ellis-Hill 2001). This may lead to mixed emotions where the carer feels resentful at being forced into a situation over which he/she has little control (Langford 1995).

It is therefore important that the family's wishes are taken into consideration when health professionals are discussing place of care and also when the patient is expressing the preferred place of death. The community palliative care clinical nurse specialist has an important role in ensuring that family members have the necessary information to make informed choices and that their voices are *heard* when discussions take place regarding the ongoing care of patients.

Care in the home

The movement away from hospital-based to community-based care has been promoted as health policy for many years, and changes such as the reduction in NHS continuing-care beds and increasing throughput of patients have had widespread impact on the community. The demand for health and social services has never been greater. The past few years have also seen many changes in the way that community nursing services are organised and how, in the absence of other nursing needs, help with personal hygiene is no longer part of the nursing role. This once core facet of nursing work has been relabelled as social care provision. The fact that health care is free and social care is chargeable and means tested adds to the problem, and many carers and family members require explanation regarding these differing services.

Case Story: Gavin

Gavin was only 46 years old and very dependent on his wife for aspects of his personal care owing to a brain tumour. His wife Ann visited the general practitioner and expressed her concerns about her ability to maintain her own employment and care for her husband. The community palliative care clinical nurse specialist was asked to visit to discuss the situation with the couple. Unfortunately, due to his age, Gavin did not qualify for free personal care from the social services; the amount payable would be means tested and dependent on their income. Gavin had considerable care needs as a result of his brain tumour, but his condition was relatively stable and was likely to need care for some months. Ann could not understand why the

---

Case Story: Gavin (*continued*)

district nursing service was unable to provide twice daily personal hygiene care for Gavin and required an explanation regarding the services. Ann eventually opted to give up her work, as paying for the care would deprive them of a considerable amount from their weekly income. The couple were referred to Welfare Rights for a further assessment of their income and possible benefits entitlements.

The largest proportion of care in the community is performed by unpaid family members, relatives, friends or even neighbours (Webb and Tossell 1999). With the shift in health policy towards the community, increased attention has been given to the needs of these carers and their caring role. Carers are predominantly women and may be the spouse, daughter or daughter-in-law of the patient; they may or may not share the same home and many will be elderly. Traditionally the caring role has been considered to be 'women's work'; however, in today's changing society that may not always be the scenario. What is known is that cancer patients, for example, spend 90% of their last year of life at home (Seale and Cartwright 1994) and that may have an enormous impact on the spouse or family member looking after the patient. Emotional strain and general disruption to their lives are common experiences for families of patients with cancer (Aoun et al. 2005).

The carer's role is shaped not only by cultural expectations, but also by the carer's own past experiences, his or her relationship with the patient and the amount of support available (Brennan 2004). Many carers find it particularly difficult to deal with incontinence and provide intimate personal care to another adult, especially when delivered to a parent. This form of role-reversal can be distressing for the carer and also the patient. It is therefore essential that health care professionals offer support to the patient's carer or carers, to enable them to sustain this vital role over what may be a protracted period of time. The community palliative care clinical nurse specialist has an important supportive role in allowing the carers to express their concerns and worries about the differing aspects of the caring role.

Practical problems

There are also many practical issues that can have a negative effect on the desirability of caring for someone at home, including the size of the house, too many people living in it, or indeed minimal space for equipment, such as a commode, hospital bed or hoist. Even today, there are some homes where the facilities may be inadequate, with shared toilets and perhaps no running hot water, for example in temporary accommodation or mobile homes. Research also suggests that areas of higher deprivation often reflect lower incomes and it may not always be financially possible for relatives to stay off work to provide care. As a direct consequence of their caring role, many carers have to reduce the hours that they work in paid employment, thereby reducing the household income. Some employers may be considerate in allowing employees time off work for their caring role or an alteration in their working hours, but sadly not all employers can be that flexible.

When there is a sick individual in the home, many extra costs are incurred which the carer may not have perceived; heating may be required 24 hours a day, prescriptions may have to be paid, extra transport costs to the hospital may be incurred and the use of the telephone may increase. It is therefore essential for the community palliative care clinical nurse specialist to assess the whole situation and liaise with the appropriate services to not only provide practical and emotional support to the patient and family, but also to maximise their income.

Case Story: Isobel

Isobel was finding life increasingly difficult. Her husband George was very unwell with pancreatic cancer. She knew the treatment was palliative, but he was undergoing chemotherapy at present and had to visit the hospital weekly. George had worked as a caretaker in the local university. His wages had never been very good, but he had been happy in his work and, with her small part-time job, they always had enough to pay the bills, etc. They had never managed to put money aside for savings. George had been off work for several months, they were living off benefits and she had struggled to continue in her part-time job. She had reluctantly given it up a few weeks previously. The cost of petrol to the hospital, the added heating and George's prescriptions were all coming out of their meagre income. Isobel was unsure how they were going to pay all the bills. The car had been bought with a hire purchase agreement and she feared they would lose the car if they could not keep up the payments. Not only was Isobel needing emotional support, but also the practical issues of their finances were her main concern. She did not feel she could give

---

Case Story: Isobel (*continued*)

all her attention to George whilst worrying about the money. The community palliative care clinical nurse specialist referred the couple to Welfare Rights for financial assistance. She also submitted a claim for a Macmillan grant to ease their immediate situation. Isobel was greatly relieved to have someone acknowledge their difficulties and give assistance. She expressed her concern that families have to carry such a burden when trying to care for their loved ones at home.

However, there are positive effects of caring for the individual at home and these include the psychological benefits of familiarity. An individual's home provides continuity, where everyone knows and understands the roles of each family member, and has a relaxing informality. It is usually a place of fond memories, happiness and security where the family feel comfortable with the surroundings and can be relaxed and gain confidence in the caring role. Many individuals derive considerable satisfaction from their caring role and are aware that they are making a positive contribution to the life of the patient (Brennan 2004). They feel a sense of achievement and relief, knowing that they have done everything possible for their loved one. Although caring for the family member at home may be a positive experience for some carers, if the caring role is extended over a long period of time it may ultimately have negative consequences on the carer in regard to health, finance and general well-being (Payne et al. 1999).

The stress of caring

Carers have always been required to care for the sick, the young, the elderly and the dying, and in many cultures these tasks are still carried out primarily by family, friends or neighbours (Payne and Ellis-Hill 2001). Indeed palliative care in the home would be impossible for many dying patients without the support of their family. Studies have regularly demonstrated that family caregivers have a variety of unmet needs, despite family support being a core aim of palliative care (Hudson 2004). As mentioned in previous chapters, palliative care is the active total care of patients and *their families* by a multiprofessional team.

In the UK the family is supported at home mainly by the community nurses and the other members of the primary health care team, along with services provided by the social work department. The primary health care team members have often known the patient prior to the illness and they will continue to care for the family afterwards (Russell and Tranter 2003). Referral to the specialist care services, usually the community palliative care clinical nurse specialist, is commonly labelled for support. However, each member of the health care team when assessing the situation may reveal differing problems and therefore working collaboratively will enhance the care and support given to the patient and family.

According to Aoun et al. (2005), research has found that families looking after patients with palliative care needs report a lack of information, communication difficulties, lack of services and lack of support as their main unmet needs. Information needs may range from knowing how to alleviate the patient's symptoms, to organising practical aids to assist in the home. Effective communication is vital to keep the carer informed about the patient, to instil confidence and to ensure the carer is well prepared for each change in the patient's deteriorating condition. It is also important for the family to ensure, through adequate assessment, that services are organised prior to a crisis occurring. Sadly, if carers do not ask for assistance they are assumed to be managing the situation and intervention may only be organised in response to a cry for help. Support from the health care professionals is therefore vitally important to sustain the situation at home, where the patient and family feel confident and well supported.

Family matters

Just as patients react differently to the diagnosis of cancer or other life-threatening illness, so do families. Illness within a household handicaps not only the individual concerned, but also the family as a whole. Their lives are disrupted and their usual family routines have to be abandoned (Langford 1995). Many spouses will also have to take on the roles traditionally undertaken by the patient, perhaps the finances, household duties or car, home and garden maintenance. The reaction and disruption within the family will depend on the illness itself and, in the case of cancer, the impact can be highly variable depending on the stage of the illness. Patients and their families often have to live through the long succession of treatments and recurrences and therefore live with uncertainty for a considerable period of time (Payne and Ellis-Hill 2001). As well as providing physical care to the patient, many carers provide the emotional support, whilst also having to cope with their own feelings of anticipated loss (Zapart et al. 2007). Caring for a sick and dying family member places heavy demands on the carers, particularly with regards to their physical, emotional and economic circumstances.

The problems can be particularly acute when the sick person has been the family breadwinner. Some women have difficulties taking on the role of the head of the household or taking over the family finances after a lifetime of being dependent (Lubkin and Payne 1998). Male carers may also find it difficult to care for their spouse, look after the children and be the sole breadwinner. These situations lead to considerable stress within the family, with limitations on family activities, social isolation and minimal respite from the caring role.

The feelings of carers may be very mixed; whilst wanting to care for their loved one, they may also feel anger, confusion, fear and a loss of control over their situation. This can at times lead to friction and frayed tempers within the family or towards the patient (Langford 1995). It may be necessary for the community palliative care clinical nurse specialist to listen to the carer and facilitate in calming a fraught situation. It may also benefit the carer if the community palliative care clinical nurse specialist explores the carer's previous experiences of caring or indeed of death within the family. They may have witnessed pain and suffering before and be anticipating this again, creating many anxieties. They may also have been *informed* by well-meaning friends or neighbours about the dying process and this may, or may not, have a bearing on reality. It will be important that the health care professionals give adequate information and reassurance to the carer about symptom control and strategies to alleviate suffering. This may relieve some of the worry and stress from the carer.

The family frequently commit to the care of their relative, giving little thought to the implications of their decision (Stajduhar and Davies 2005). Few carers will have any idea of the major impact the caring role will have on their own lives. The agreement to care for the loved one at home may have been made early on in the illness trajectory and the family feel obliged to honour that decision. Alternatively it may be made when the patient is nearing death and in hospital; perceived pressure may be felt by the family to comply, because the patient is desperate for home. Many of these decisions are made by the family who are expecting the caregiving time to be short due to the patient's weakening condition. However, they may not have given any thought to the situation should it extend beyond a few days or weeks (Stajduhar and Davies 2005). Many caregivers are determined to keep promises that have been made to the patient, even when the care becomes hard to manage and the carer has difficulty sustaining the situation. This may result in feelings of guilt when carers realise they can no longer cope, particularly if the patient subsequently requires end-of-life care in a hospice or hospital setting. Carers therefore need to express their complex feelings and be aware that non-judgemental support is available.

Physical demands

Difficulty sleeping and poor appetite are also reported by carers. They find that their whole day and at times their nights are consumed in caring for the patient, particularly as death approaches, leaving little time for sleep or cooking a meal. Feeling continually tired can be one of the most challenging disruptions for carers and, compounded with their erratic eating patterns, their energy levels may soon start to diminish. The carer's disturbed sleep patterns, resulting from 24-hour caregiving, soon contribute to stress and exhaustion (Hearson and McClement 2007). Sleep disturbance has a physical effect but also psychological repercussions and may lead to increasing feelings of isolation (Rose 2001). Helpful enquiries about the welfare of the carer will elicit these problems and allow them to be addressed. The offer of Marie Curie nurses to sit with the patient overnight may be useful and allow the carer to have a night's rest. Organisations such as the Crossroads Care Attendant Scheme can give carers respite for a few hours, to permit them to go shopping or simply take a break from caring.

It is, however, dependent on the health care professional, often the community palliative care clinical nurse specialist, developing a comfortable, trusting relationship with carers and permitting them to express their needs, emotions, anxieties and complex problems. Carers may also have feelings of guilt for what appears to be bemoaning their own situation, especially when their loved one is very ill or dying. Again it is incumbent on the community palliative care clinical nurse specialist to inform the carer that these emotions are normal and offer support and reassurance to the carer and family at this distressing time.

Case Story: Sarah

Sarah's mother was a widow and had cared for Sarah since her diagnosis of oesophageal cancer some months previously. Sarah wanted to die at home with her mum and, despite her mother's frailty, mum had agreed that she would care for her daughter. Mum adamantly

---

Case Story: Sarah (*continued*)

refused help from any of the services and coped well with feeding Sarah through a PEG tube, her medication administration, multiple episodes of haemorrhaging from the tumour and many sleepless nights. However, the endless climbing of the stairs, washing bed-linen and keeping the house, as well as the nursing care of Sarah, was taking its toll on mum. She began to lose weight and looked exhausted. The community palliative care clinical nurse specialist feared that Sarah's mother may be unable to continue caring for Sarah until her death, because of her own deteriorating health. When offered help Sarah's mother refused and became very upset, reporting that she would be letting Sarah down if she had to accept assistance with her care. The community palliative care clinical nurse specialist explained to Sarah's mother her concerns about the situation, explaining that the health care professionals wanted to support her in her efforts to care for Sarah and not take over the care of her daughter. After a lot of tears and sobbing, Sarah's mother expressed her own anxieties; she admitted having had little sleep for several weeks and very little to eat due to the demands of the caring role. She expressed guilt at having to ask for help when it was her own daughter who was dying. It was agreed that social services would be asked for assistance with the household tasks such as laundry and Marie Curie nurses would provide some night cover to allow Sarah's mother to rest. Sarah died at home, but the caring role had been difficult for her mother. She admitted afterwards that when Sarah had asked to die at home her response had been automatic and she would not have considered anything else at the time. However, she reported that, with hindsight, it had been much more difficult than she had ever imagined and she should have accepted help at an earlier stage.

Many family carers carry out complex nursing care to very ill individuals and where the illness follows a progressive course they get little relief and are continually required to adapt and change according to the demands of the illness. Caring can be hard work physically and it is easy for the health care professionals to overlook the difficulties that family carers may have with basic nursing tasks, for example, helping someone to dress, sitting the patient up in bed, personal hygiene needs, including hair care and oral hygiene, toileting and transferring between bed and commode (Rose 2001). Carers are not prepared for these tasks and often learn by trial and error.

The physical environment where the care takes place (usually the patient's home) can in itself cause stress and problems for the carer. Private houses were never designed as places where the sick would be cared for and nursed until death. Many homes have two storeys and, if the patient is upstairs, then the carer may be climbing the stairs many times a day – no easy task for an elderly carer. It may not always be possible to make room for a hospital bed within the home and a carer may have to struggle giving nursing care and assistance to the patient in a large double bed. Bathrooms and toilets are rarely built with thought of possible wheelchair use, nor household baths constructed to allow the less mobile patient to get in and out safely and with ease. These problems will only add to the frustration and anxiety that most carers feel in their own particular situation. As a result of the physical difficulties, the feelings of frustration and loss of control that the patient may also be experiencing can be directed towards the carer as anger or impatience.

All these problems have to be addressed and solutions found to lessen the distress on the carer. The community palliative care clinical nurse specialist may spend considerable time with the carer identifying complex problems and then making referrals to the occupational therapist for assistance regarding the physical environment, or to the social services for assistance with the patient's personal hygiene.

The burden of caring

Carers feel an immense sense of responsibility towards their loved ones in terms of their physical well-being, deciding when to seek medical treatment, and what medications to administer and when. They need constant reassurance, information and support in their capacity as the main carer. Even the day-to-day household decisions that many take for granted can cause anxiety and upset.

Case Story: Martin

Martin was in the last few weeks of life and being cared for at home by his wife. She found the caring role exhausting and frustrating. However, Martin had expressed a desire to die at home and his wife was determined to fulfil his wishes. The community palliative care clinical nurse specialist was visiting regularly to support the couple and had organised considerable help for them. She received a telephone

---

Case Story: Martin (*continued*)

call one day from Martin's wife; she was very distressed and wanted the community palliative care clinical nurse specialist to come immediately. Fearing the worst, a likely change in Martin's condition, the nurse cancelled another visit and went straight to their house. When she arrived, Martin's wife was sobbing and very distressed and it took several minutes to work out the problem. Martin's wife wanted to know what she could give Martin for his lunch as he reported being hungry, but she had reached the end of her resources in trying to tempt his appetite. This was a symptom of her overall stress and she had reached the end of her coping abilities. The community palliative care clinical nurse specialist discussed the situation with the couple and it was agreed that Martin's daughter would come and care for her father for a few days and his wife would go to their son for a break. After 3 days Martin's wife returned feeling more relaxed and once again able to care for her husband.

It is not uncommon for carers to feel overwhelmed by their situation. However, due to the demands of the caring role, their own health needs are often given a lower priority than the patient. This may result in situations, as demonstrated in the above scenario, where the carer reaches his or her limits. A study conducted by Zapart et al. (2007) found that carers worked greater than 11 hours a day directly providing care to the patient, and it is therefore not surprising that carers also report a knock-on effect on their emotional and mental health. It is important for the health care professionals involved in the patient's care, especially the community palliative care clinical nurse specialist, to identify when the carer is becoming exhausted and act to avert a crisis. Respite care should be on offer to carers; this may be as overnight care, a few hours per week or more regularly as needs arise. Families often decline offers of respite, believing that they will manage, but it is important that they understand the significance of respite breaks. It may need to be explained to the family that the professionals are there to help care for the patient and not to *take over* the care of the loved one. The community palliative care clinical nurse specialist is skilled in listening to carers and encouraging them to express their complex anxieties and give emotional support, but also to impart practical information and advice to prepare and assist carers in this demanding role.

Social isolation can have a negative effect on the carer's emotional state. Many carers find that the relationships with their friends change, and this may be for a variety of reasons. They may be unable to get out socially because the patient cannot be left alone, or the loved one expresses a desire to have the carer around all the time. There is a loss of spontaneity in the carer's everyday life and the daily routine revolves around, and is dictated by, the patient and his or her care. Feelings of guilt may manifest if the carer tries to go out shopping or leaves the patient with someone else, even for a brief time.

Case Story: Terry

Terry was very unwell with myeloma and nearing the end of his life. His wife Anna was very tired and had few family or friends to support her in the caring role. Terry became agitated and upset whenever she left the room and he would not hear of anyone else staying with him. This had been the scenario for 3 weeks and Anna was finding it increasingly difficult to meet his demands. In that time, she had not been out of the house for shopping or even to walk around the garden for fresh air. She was starting to express anger at Terry and reported to the community palliative care clinical nurse specialist that Terry had never been demanding in their 30 years together, but now she thought his behaviour very selfish. She also felt very guilty at saying these things about her husband when he was so close to death. Anna was encouraged to vent her mixed feelings and also explore possible solutions to the problem. It was very difficult to talk to Anna as Terry shouted for her attention constantly. The community palliative care clinical nurse specialist facilitated a discussion between Anna and Terry and with some prompting both expressed their complex emotions. Terry admitted to fear and wanting Anna to be with him at the moment of death; he was frightened that if she left the room he might die without her present. Anna reported being very aware of his changing condition and that when death was imminent she would be there, but, for now, she needed a little space to rest and recuperate her strength. Terry reluctantly agreed that Anna should have an hour each afternoon for herself and they organised a rota from the limited family and friends to be with Terry. He was informed that Anna would never be too far away and would always have her mobile telephone with her. Terry did in fact settle when she was away and found he could enjoy the company of someone else for

---

Case Story: Terry (*continued*)

an hour. However, Anna always had to be back in exactly an hour or Terry started to fret again. Anna found the hour was never enough, but continued for a further 10 days until Terry deteriorated and died with Anna present.

Brennan (2004) reports that the relationship between the carer and the patient is an important factor in determining the level of stress the carer will experience. Stress is more likely where the patient refuses the help being offered, if the patient is very negative and expects too much of the carer, or where the patient constantly makes demands on the carer. In research undertaken by Eriksson and Svedlund (2006) carers described their ill spouses as altering in character and becoming increasingly self-centred. This may be particularly difficult for a couple who have been loving and considerate to each other for many years. The physical relationship between the patient and spouse may also change as a result of the illness. A lack of intimacy, altered sexual relationships and feelings of loneliness may be experienced, even when living together as a couple; unfortunately some spouses see themselves more as a care provider than as a wife or husband (Eriksson and Svedlund 2006). This can bring sadness and feelings of emptiness. Carers need to express their feelings, as an inability to vent these emotions may lead to a rise in anger and a sense of helplessness (Redgrove and Smyth 2000). The carer may at times suffer from more emotional distress than the patient. It is therefore important that psychological and emotional help is directed specifically at the carer, with the community palliative care clinical nurse specialist having the skills and experience to provide the support needed.

Supporting the carers

Nurses hold a unique position among health care providers in terms of prolonged contact with patients and their families whilst they are being cared for at home. This may be from the district nursing service who will be providing the hands-on physical care to the patient, or indeed the community palliative care clinical nurse specialist who will be addressing the complicated psychosocial needs of the patient and family, as well as possible complex symptom control issues. The patient's illness trajectory may extend over many months or years and the community palliative care clinical nurse specialist will become familiar with the family during that time, whether contact has been sporadic, as problems arise, or continuous due to complex and difficult problems. During contacts the community palliative care clinical nurse specialist will have identified the support structure within the family, the carer's previous experience of the caring role, any history of mental health problems, evidence of poor coping skills or dependency on drugs or alcohol. Consideration and regard for the carer has an important preventive health element, as both the future physical and mental health of the carer can be influenced partly by his or her experience of the dying patient's illness and death (Monroe and Sheldon 2004).

Information needs

The role of the community palliative care clinical nurse specialist involves intervention with families and carers to promote their coping skills. This may be where there are complex and difficult emotional, family or other problems to be addressed. The detailed assessment of the family and carer can identify individuals who may be at particular risk and will benefit from increased support (Monroe and Sheldon 2004). To assist the family to make choices and feel empowered, the community palliative care clinical nurse specialist needs to assess the knowledge base of the individuals, provide information and advice as required and ensure that there is full understanding of the situation. Carers need to be told what the caring role will involve, the probable course of the illness and what support is available to them (Brennan 2004). There is a great need to ensure families have adequate information and are taught the practical aspects of care so that they can make informed decisions about taking on the care at home.

Case Story: Lorna

Lorna was in the local hospital recovering from surgery for an advanced bowel cancer. She was aware that time was now limited but wanted to go home for her final few weeks. Her husband had many anxieties about caring for her, not least looking after her stoma and the urinary catheter. The hospital palliative care team had visited Lorna and resolved her physical symptoms of pain and nausea and

---

Case Story: Lorna (*continued*)

felt she was ready for home. They had spoken to her husband on many occasions, but he had always found more barriers to her going home. The community palliative care clinical nurse specialist had met the couple prior to Lorna's admission for surgery and was asked by the hospital team to visit Lorna's husband at home to discuss his fears and anxieties. The community palliative care clinical nurse specialist visited Lorna's husband, with Lorna's consent, accompanied by the district nurse, to discuss the practicalities of Lorna going home. After a long discussion, where many doubts were expressed by Lorna's husband about his ability to cope, it was agreed that Lorna would come home. Her husband had been reassured by the additional practical information about caring for the stoma and also care of the urinary catheter, as well as the offers of practical help from the district nursing service. He now felt he had a greater knowledge of what practical care Lorna would need and where to seek help if difficulties arose.

In many instances, the general practitioner, district nurse or hospital palliative care team may ask the community palliative care clinical nurse specialist to visit the family at home, to discuss the many facets of the caring role and the complex practical and emotional issues that may ensue. The purpose of addressing potential problems is to allow the family or carer to discuss issues and determine possible solutions in advance, knowing what help is available, rather than the professionals having to intervene when a crisis ensues. A family-solved problem has a greater likelihood of success than one that the professionals have proposed or inflicted on the family. The carer and family need to be given the opportunity to express their concerns and verbalise the worst and best aspects of caring for their loved one. They require knowing where help can be obtained 24 hours a day, what changes can be expected in the patient's condition and the practicalities of nursing care, such as medication administration. The family's need for written and verbal information may be considerable and the community palliative care clinical nurse specialist may have to invest significant time and resources to ensure the family feel adequately informed.

The community palliative care clinical nurse specialist will also need to assess the understanding of the carer and utilise vocabulary and linguistic style appropriate to each individual (Monroe and

Sheldon 2004). The family may require time and the opportunity to ask questions, to have information repeated and to verbalise any issues with which they still have doubts or misgivings. Effective communication is the key to success in caring for the patient at home and the community palliative care clinical nurse specialist should use her skills, knowledge and expertise to keep the family abreast of the patient's situation at all times.

Case Story: Jethro

Jethro's family were very caring and happy to have him at home for the remainder of his life. They had considerable information needs regarding his disease, his deterioration, his care and how to care for him emotionally. When the palliative care clinical nurse specialist visited Jethro she knew that her visit to the patient would be brief; Jethro rarely asked questions, appeared accepting of his situation and always seemed contented. However, his family would want to talk to the community palliative care clinical nurse specialist for long periods of time. They had many questions, some technical regarding the disease process and others of a more practical nature relating to his care. The community palliative care clinical nurse specialist always allocated significant time to sit with the family and address their information needs. It allowed them to feel more in control of the situation and acknowledged the importance of their contribution to Jethro's care.

Practical needs

Support to carers may take many forms, depending on the individual situation. As discussed previously, carers may ask for help within the home to assist with the household duties. It is therefore important to refer on to social services when necessary or indeed for the family to be informed about private agencies that may provide help with tasks around the home. It should be noted, however, that the various providers, i.e. health, social care, private agencies, etc., will create a continuous stream of people through the patient's house and this may be looked upon as an intrusion; therefore a balance has to be achieved where assistance is being provided, but the patient and family maintain their privacy.

For many individuals and their family, the financial situation may be of the greatest concern. When there is insufficient income to pay the monthly accounts, etc., considerable stress may develop within the household. This only adds to the burden on the carer and causes undue worry for the patient. Again it may be incumbent on the community palliative care clinical nurse specialist to refer on to the appropriate agencies, such as Welfare Rights or the Citizens Advice Bureau, to assess the family income and maximise their resources. Carers are often elderly and may be frail themselves; therefore it is necessary to assess their physical and emotional ability to take on the caring role. They may require considerable support – both practical and emotional; many will verbalise their fears of being alone after a lifetime with their loved one.

Case Story: Rita

Rita was dying from breast cancer. She was 83 years of age and had a son who lived nearby. Her husband (86) had traditionally been the breadwinner in the home; he had worked as a motor mechanic all his working years, he tended the garden, looked after their car and maintained the house. He had never in their 58 years of marriage cooked a meal, washed the dishes or undertaken any housework. He knew nothing about the finances, the complexity of the washing machine or how to iron a shirt. Rita informed the community palliative care clinical nurse specialist that they had had a good marriage where each played their part and it had always worked well. However, she was now very worried about how he would manage to care for himself after her death. Her husband was bereft at the thought of Rita not being there for him, she had always been his companion and friend. Rita's son and daughter-in-law promised to take care of Rita's husband and provide as much assistance as he required until he was able to manage on his own. After Rita's death, her husband required considerable emotional and practical support not only from the family, but also from the health and social services.

The emotional support required by carers of all ages may be significant. Children's needs also have to be given consideration as they may be watching a parent or grandparent dying and may be feeling lost and bewildered by the whole situation. They require time and the opportunity to express their emotions; this may be together with the patient or alone with the professional. Many of the carers, whatever their age, will not want their loved one to see their distress and will appreciate time with the community palliative care clinical nurse specialist to vent their feelings. Carers will see the patient as vulnerable and may want to protect him or her and therefore may not share their fears and emotions with their loved one (Ellis-Hill 2001). Zapart et al. (2007) report that carers find it difficult to cope with the patient in pain, crying or upset. Therefore carers need the opportunity to relate this to a professional who has time, knowledge and skills to manage their emotional distress.

The community palliative care clinical nurse specialist will also require knowledge of the cultural beliefs and social expectations of the individual and family. In some cultures a chronic illness may be seen as a form of punishment for previous wrong-doing and this perception can influence the family's response to the patient and his or her illness. It is therefore important for the community palliative care clinical nurse specialist to effectively communicate with the family to ensure an understanding of their own particular situation and offer support appropriately.

Carers as co-workers

According to Eriksson and Svedlund (2006), many families feel neglected and their needs are underestimated by the professionals. Attention tends to focus on the patient and the needs of the carer may not always be adequately recognised (Langford 1995). There requires to be recognition and valuing of the role of carers from the health care professionals and carers need to be informed that they are co-workers in the patient's care and of the importance of their contribution. This can do much to bolster the confidence of carers and enable them to continue caring when they face difficulties.

Assessing the needs of the carer should be a priority when health care professionals visit the household. Addressing only the patient's needs may leave the carer practically and emotionally bereft, as well as neglected and undervalued. It has to be remembered that many of these carers will be providing care 24 hours a day and that will include many tasks such as washing, cleaning dentures, feeding, toileting, emptying commodes, lifting, turning and transferring, as well as administration of medications and dealing with ongoing symptoms. Whilst some carers can learn these new skills easily, others may worry about the responsibility and resent the intrusion and subtle changes they bring into the relationship with their loved one (Payne and Ellis-Hill 2001). Many will find some of the tasks difficult, such as emptying a commode, and, knowing that this is not a single occurrence but an ongoing situation, they may find it emotionally demanding (Rose 2001).

Hence the need for carers to express their feelings and the health care professionals to offer support in whatever way possible. As well as offering an opportunity to carers to express their emotions, the community palliative care clinical nurse specialist may introduce simple strategies such as prescription charts, dosette boxes for medications, advice on symptoms or organising useful pieces of equipment to assist the carer. Fatigue and lack of sleep commonly affect carers; this can impact on their competence and confidence in the caring role (Hearson and McClement 2007). Carers cannot sustain the caring role for 24 hours a day for long periods without a break; however, many will feel guilty if they take time out. The community palliative clinical nurse specialist can listen to the complex emotions of carers and explain that their feelings are normal and that respite for a few hours will enhance their ability to perform the caring role.

For many carers, it is assumed that the assistance they require would be in caring directly for the patient, i.e. bathing, toileting, etc., but in fact what they often need is someone to peel the potatoes, prepare the family meals, run errands, walk the dog and generally help around the house. Sadly few services within the present health or social sector provide this broad type of care and it often has to be sought from the private sector.

Case Story: Peter

Peter had lung cancer with brain metastases. His wife found the everyday caring of Peter difficult, but the requirement for help within the home was an even greater need. She had Marie Curie nurses and social services assisting with Peter's personal care, but continually felt they would be more productive if they allowed her to care for Peter and the help was targeted at washing the dirty dishes, preparing the evening meal or cutting the grass. These were chores that she found not only increasingly difficult, but also time consuming, and she could not understand why the nurses and helpers were unable to undertake these domestic activities. This caused continual strife between Peter's wife and the professionals for the duration of his illness. The community palliative care clinical nurse specialist organised a meeting with the professionals involved in Peter's care. With reflection, they reported that perhaps the help was targeted at where the professionals felt there was a need, i.e. in caring for the patient, instead of caring for the carer. By allowing his wife to provide Peter's personal care and targeting the help at her needs, the situation could have been immensely improved. This would have allowed Peter and his wife quality time together and considerably less anxiety for his wife.

The findings of a study by Zapart et al. (2007) support the view that carers needs are often practical in nature and include meal preparation and assistance with general housework, whilst a previous study by Perreault et al. (2004) also identified that the best support to carers was when friends provided practical help such as cooking a meal or doing the housekeeping. The role of the community palliative care clinical nurse specialist is therefore to ensure that the carer and family's complex needs are being addressed, as well as that of the patient. Liaison with the other health care professionals and the social services should be aimed at maximising the support for the family in a practical way and also providing the emotional support to minimise the distress and anxiety.

When the disease begins to progress, carers may experience increasing feelings of loss. If they have been able to continue with their paid employment during the previous weeks or months of the patient's illness, they may now have to cease working. They will lose contact with work colleagues, friends and acquaintances as their lives become consumed by the caring role. Social isolation ensues and therefore it is important that they are given every opportunity to express their emotions at this time. Carers will appreciate knowing that the health care professionals care about what is happening to them (Langford 1995). Telephone contact and visits to the home by the community palliative care clinical nurse specialist can give the support that the carer needs at this time.

Approaching death

In the past, families were more familiar with illness and death at home; however, today many will have had no previous experience in caring for someone who is dying, let alone the death of a loved one. As the patient's condition deteriorates and death approaches, the carer and family may request information about the dying process and death itself. The community palliative care clinical nurse specialist may be using her skills in teaching, advising and encouraging the carer in this frightening new role. Sensitivity is required when discussing the subject and, in particular, caution should be used until it is ascertained whether all parties are ready to discuss this emotional subject. The community palliative care clinical nurse specialist will be able to utilise her experience and extensive knowledge in dealing with these requests and providing information in a sensitive manner. Carers may need some time and encouragement to express their worries about death and to feel that they are being supported in the final stages of the patient's life. They may have concerns about possible symptoms they associate with death such as pain, confusion, incontinence or loss of consciousness. The community palliative care clinical nurse specialist can take time to explore these issues and discuss simple strategies for the carer to adopt should difficulties arise and also when to seek assistance.

For some individuals, the dying process may be prolonged, and as a result of the stress of caring for the patient and waiting for the imminent death, the carer and family may become exhausted and emotionally drained. The last hours may not be the peaceful, calm scenario depicted in the movies; instead there may be family strife or relatives in attendance who have not spoken to each other for many years. The health care professionals may encounter considerable friction between family members and at times a rivalry within the family over who should act as the main carer (Langford 1995). The community palliative care clinical nurse specialist may have to listen to all their concerns and emotional issues, whilst remembering that the display of strong feelings at this time may cause further conflict or upset to others. The support required by the carer and family at this time may be considerable. Many carers are frightened at the prospect of the death and of their own reactions once the death has occurred, such as panic or overwhelming distress. They may need significant reassurance and an opportunity to voice these fears. It needs to be explained to the carer and family that even when expected, the death of their loved one will come as a profound emotional and often physical shock (Monroe and Sheldon 2004). The health care professionals involved in the patient's care need to ensure that the family have been informed about what to do after the death, particularly if this happens out-of-hours when their own general practitioner's surgery is closed.

Caring for dying patients and their families requires a multidisciplinary approach. The health care professionals involved should all work collaboratively to ensure that the needs of the patient and their family are achieved in a caring and sensitive manner. The community palliative care clinical nurse specialist may be heavily involved with the family and giving considerable support. A trusting therapeutic relationship may have developed over many months, or indeed years, when the family or patient may have required specialist intervention at different times during the illness, for a variety of complex problems. There may also be occasions where the community palliative care clinical nurse specialist may not have direct contact with the patient or carer; however, advice may be sought from another member of the primary health care team on issues such as complex psychosocial support or unresolved symptom control. It is therefore incumbent on the community palliative care clinical nurse specialist to ensure that the other health care professionals are aware of the role of the specialist nurse, reasons for referral and how to refer. The advice or intervention from the community palliative care clinical nurse specialist can be invaluable in improving the quality of life of carers in the community setting (Langford 1995).

Key Points

- Family members and informal carers are the single most important resource for looking after patients at home with a long-term or life-threatening illness.
- The carer and family will experience numerous losses as a result of their loved ones diagnosis and these may include loss of future plans, loss of being an *ordinary* family and a loss of freedom.
- Many families agree to look after their loved one at home because that is what the patient has requested; however, the family may have little insight into the caring role and the significant implications for the whole family.
- The community palliative care clinical nurse specialist has an important role in ensuring that family members have the necessary information to make informed choices and that their voices are *heard* when discussions take place regarding the ongoing care of patients.
- Caring for a sick and dying family member places heavy demands on the carers, particularly with regards to their physical, emotional and economic circumstances.
- Many family carers carry out complex nursing care to very ill individuals and where the illness follows a progressive course they get little relief and are continually required to adapt and change according to the demands of the illness.

Key Points (*continued*)

- The community palliative care clinical nurse specialist is skilled in listening to carers, encouraging them to express their complex anxieties and giving emotional support, but also in imparting practical information and advice to prepare and assist carers in this demanding role.
- To assist the family to make choices and feel empowered, the community palliative care clinical nurse specialist needs to assess the knowledge base of the individuals, provide information and advice as required and ensure that there is full understanding of the situation.
- There requires to be recognition and valuing of the role of carers from the health care professionals and carers need to be informed that they are co-workers in the patient's care and of the importance of their contribution.

Useful resources

Aoun SM, Kristjanson LJ, Currow DC, Hudson PL (2005) Caregiving for the terminally ill: at what cost? *Palliative Medicine* 19 (7), 551–555.

Brennan J (2004) *Cancer in Context: A Practical Guide to Supportive Care.* Oxford University Press, Oxford.

Eriksson M, Svedlund M (2006) The intruder: spouses' narratives about life with a chronically ill partner. *Journal of Clinical Nursing* 15 (3), 324–333.

Hearson B, McClement S (2007) Sleep disturbance in family caregivers of patients with advanced cancer. *International Journal of Palliative Nursing* 13 (10), 495–501.

Payne S, Ellis-Hill C (eds) (2001) *Chronic and Terminal Illness: New Perspectives on Caring and Carers.* Oxford University Press, Oxford.

Perreault A, Fothergill-Bourbonnais F, Fiset V (2004) The experience of family members caring for a dying loved one. *International Journal of Palliative Nursing* 10 (3), 133–143.

Stajduhar KI, Davies B (2005) Variations in and factors influencing family members' decisions for palliative home care. *Palliative Medicine* 19 (1), 21–32.

References

Altschuler J, Dale B, Byng-Hall J (1997) *Working with Chronic Illness.* Macmillan, Basingstoke.

Aoun SM, Kristjanson LJ, Currow DC, Hudson PL (2005) Caregiving for the terminally ill: at what cost? *Palliative Medicine* 19 (7), 551–555.

Brennan J (2004) *Cancer in Context: A Practical Guide to Supportive Care.* Oxford University Press, Oxford.

Coote A (1996) Options for long term care. In: Harding T, Meredith B, Wistow G (eds) (1996) *Options for Long Term Care*, pp 99–106. HMSO, London.

Edwards NE, Scheetz PS (2002) Predictors of burden for caregivers of patients with Parkinson's disease. *Journal of Neuroscience Nursing* 34 (4), 184–190.

Ellis-Hill C (2001) Caring and identity: the experience of spouses in stroke and other chronic neurological conditions. In: Payne S, Ellis-Hill C (eds) *Chronic and Terminal Illness: New Perspectives on Caring and Carers*, pp 44–63. Oxford University Press, Oxford.

Eriksson M, Svedlund M (2006) The intruder: spouses' narratives about life with a chronically ill partner. *Journal of Clinical Nursing* 15 (3), 324–333.

Greenberg JS, Boyd MD, Hale JF (1992) *The Caregiver's Guide: For Caregivers and the Elderly.* Nelson-Hall, Chicago.

Hearson B, McClement S (2007) Sleep disturbance in family caregivers of patients with advanced cancer. *International Journal of Palliative Nursing* 13 (10), 495–501.

Hudson P (2004) Positive aspects and challenges associated with caring for a dying relative at home. *International Journal of Palliative Nursing* 10 (2), 58–64.

Langford L (1995) Care in the home. In: Robbins J, Moscrop J (eds) *Caring for the Dying Patient and the Family*, 3rd edn, pp 208–222. Chapman and Hall, London.

Lubkin I, Payne ME (1998) Family caregivers. In: Lubkin IM, Larsen PD (eds) *Chronic Illness: Impact and Interventions*, 4th edn, pp 258–282. Jones and Bartlett, Sudbury.

Monroe B, Sheldon F (2004) Psychosocial dimensions of care. In: Sykes N, Edmonds P, Wiles J (eds) *Management of Advanced Disease*, pp 405–437. Arnold, London.

Payne S, Ellis-Hill C (eds) (2001) *Chronic and Terminal Illness: New Perspectives on Caring and Carers.* Oxford University Press, Oxford.

Payne S, Smith P, Dean S (1999) Identifying the concerns of informal carers in palliative care. *Palliative Medicine* 13 (1), 37–44.

Perreault A, Fothergill-Bourbonnais F, Fiset V (2004) The experience of family members caring for a dying loved one. *International Journal of Palliative Nursing* 10 (3), 133–143.

Redgrove M, Smyth A (2000) Hearing the pain of the carer. In: Cooper J (ed) *Stepping into Palliative Care: A Handbook for Community Professionals*, pp 119–125. Radcliffe Medical Press, Abingdon.

Rose K (2001) A longitudinal study of carers providing palliative care. In: Payne S, Ellis-Hill C (eds) *Chronic and Terminal Illness: New Perspectives on Caring and Carers*, pp 64–82. Oxford University Press, Oxford.

Russell D, Tranter G (2003) Organisation of palliative care services. In: Gore M, Russell D (eds) *Cancer in Primary Care*, pp 17–20. Martin Dunitz, London.

Seale C, Cartwright A (1994) *The Year Before Death*. Avebury, Aldershot.

Smith P (2001) Who is a carer? Experiences of family caregivers in palliative care. In: Payne S, Ellis-Hill C (eds) *Chronic and Terminal Illness: New Perspectives on Caring and Carers*, pp 83–99. Oxford University Press, Oxford.

Stajduhar KI, Davies B (2005) Variations in and factors influencing family members' decisions for palliative home care. *Palliative Medicine* 19 (1), 21–32.

Webb R, Tossell D (1999) *Social Issues for Carers: Towards Positive Practice*, 2nd edn. Arnold, London.

Zapart S, Kenny P, Hall J, Servis B, Wiley S (2007) Home-based palliative care in Sydney, Australia: the carer's perspective on the provision of informal care. *Health and Social Care in the Community* 15 (2), 97–107.

Loss and Bereavement

Introduction

The death of a loved individual is an experience that everybody confronts at some point in life. This loss brings emotional pain and grief to the bereaved and can be described as the most severe psychological trauma people will encounter in their lives (Parkes and Weiss 1983). The grief experienced may be mild or severe, it may be short-lived or protracted, it may have an immediate onset or, for some people, a delayed onset (Parkes 1998). Grief changes individuals and their families, as life will never be quite the same again (Doyle and Jeffrey 2000).

Bereavement is associated with mental and physical health problems (Stroebe et al. 2003). This results in a high mortality within the bereaved population and up to a third of bereaved individuals developing a depressive illness (Sheldon 1998). However, bereavement has become a topic with which people are uncomfortable and death is a subject that society avoids (Main 2002). Recent demographic changes and patterns of disease have had an effect on people's experiences of dying and on the sources of support available to patients and their families (Seale 2001). The erosion of the extended family and the disregard of formal mourning have meant that the bereaved get little support from their families or society. Many of the rituals associated with death have disappeared, leaving bereaved individuals isolated and often confused about their feelings (Kindlen et al. 1999).

Melliar-Smith (2002) describes bereavement support as incorporating the understanding and recognition of an individual's grief and his or her need for psychological support. One of the elements of palliative care is the provision of support in bereavement; therefore the nursing care and responsibilities to dying patients and their families do not end with the death of the patient (Matzo et al. 2003). Primary care health professionals are ideally placed to provide bereavement assessment and subsequent interventions. The community palliative care clinical nurse specialist is in a unique position to be able to offer support to families, not only during a patient's illness and death, but also into the bereavement period. As a patient's condition deteriorates, more time and effort can be spent supporting the carers, helping them begin their grieving and preparing them for the death. The role of the community palliative care clinical nurse specialist includes facilitating the grief process by assessing grief, assisting the survivor to feel and express the loss and helping the bereaved to work through the stages of grief.

Grief and loss

According to Stroebe et al. (1993), grief is not only a complex syndrome, but also a natural phenomenon with diverse outcomes. Reactions described by many authors on the subject include feelings of sadness, anger, guilt, anxiety, loneliness, fatigue, helplessness, shock, yearning, relief, numbness and restlessness (Raphael 1985; Worden 1991; Wright 1991; Corr et al. 2003). One of the most characteristic features of grief described by Parkes (1998) is acute and episodic *pangs*; this is an episode of anxiety and psychological pain which can begin within hours or days of bereavement and usually peaks within 5–14 days. This may be accompanied by crying and the bereaved searching for the deceased loved one. Corr et al. (2003) also describe behaviours that may manifest, such as sleep or appetite disturbances, forgetfulness, social withdrawal, dreams of the deceased, avoiding reminders of the deceased, searching and calling out, restless overactivity or visiting places that remind the bereaved of the deceased.

The seminal work by Lindemann (1944), a pioneer in the field of grief, described physical sensations of grief including hollowness in the stomach, tightness in the chest and throat, dry mouth, breathlessness and general weakness. These sensations may occur in waves and last from 20–60 minutes, though not all bereaved individuals will experience or report these physical manifestations. For some, these physical symptoms may result from anxiety and can also mimic the symptoms experienced by the deceased. It is important for the health care professionals, however, to be aware of these physical sensations as they are at times overlooked, but do play a significant role in the grieving process. They may be of great concern to bereaved people who subsequently

visit the general practitioner believing that they may themselves be
seriously ill.

Case Story: Colin

Colin's wife of 22 years had died recently from lung cancer. Colin
felt that he was coping relatively well with the bereavement and had
managed to go back to work. However, he had visited the general
practitioner several times complaining of tiredness and was now
experiencing some chest tightness at rest. The general practitioner
had discussed Colin's symptoms with him and they agreed not to do
any invasive investigations at present. The community palliative care
clinical nurse specialist was due to visit Colin at home and had been
updated by the GP on Colin's consultations. During the visit Colin
discussed at length his symptoms and their similarity to those experienced by his wife at the start of her illness. He required reassurance
and support to express his emotions and concerns at this time. Over
a few weeks his symptoms gradually settled and he realised that he
did not have a serious physical illness.

Although most individuals possess adequate resources to cope
with bereavement, for some the challenge can be difficult (Woof and
Nyatanga 1998). The term *bereavement* refers to the state of being
bereaved or robbed of something (Corr et al. 2003). This usually relates
to the loss of a person to whom the bereaved has had an attachment.
Grief is the personal reaction to the loss, both psychological and emotional, and *mourning* is the public display of that loss (Steen 1998). There
are a number of theoretical frameworks in the literature that describe
the reactions and experiences of bereavement and these may assist
health care professionals to understand reactions to grief.

Theoretical frameworks

Grief was described by Lindemann (1944) as a definite syndrome with
psychological and somatic symptomatology. Factors included in this
syndrome are somatic distress, preoccupation with the image of the
deceased, guilt and hostile reactions. He reported that this syndrome
might appear immediately after a crisis, it may be delayed, it may be
overstated or absent. He also found that the picture shown by persons

in grief was remarkably uniform and suggested that to a certain extent the pattern and severity of the reaction can be predicted. Kubler-Ross (1969) described stages of dying; this has subsequently been applied to bereavement. She described a five-stage model: denial, anger, bargaining, depression and acceptance. Bowlby (1981) wrote extensively about attachment and loss and he suggests that when attachment bonds are broken, behaviours such as clinging, crying, anger and protest are activated. Bowlby describes four phases of mourning: a phase of numbness which may last hours to weeks; a phase of yearning and searching which can continue for months or years; a phase of disorganisation and despair; and finally a phase of reorganisation.

Stroebe and Stroebe (1987) report that the initial response to bereavement is shock, numbness and disbelief. They suggest this may be broken by bursts of anger or despair. After the initial numbness, periods of strong emotions ensue with psychological distress as the awareness of the loss develops. They report that a feature of this stage is the tendency to search for the deceased. Through time, the searching is abandoned and the loss is gradually recognised. This can be when apathy and depression develop and the process of overcoming these can be slow. They report that for most people, the negative reactions and emotions begin to be interspersed by more positive and less devastating reactions. Worden (1991) states that it is necessary for the bereaved to accomplish certain *tasks* of mourning: the first task is to accept the loss and acknowledge that the person will not return; the second is to work through the pain of grief; and the third is to adjust to an environment without the deceased. The final task is to emotionally relocate the deceased and move on with life. He reports that a completed grief reaction is when the person is able to think about the deceased without pain.

Parkes (1998) describes grief as a process and not a state. He explains that grief is not a set of symptoms, which start after a loss and then fade, but a series of phases, each with its own characteristics. He defines four phases of grieving, but he suggests that there are considerable differences from person to person. His first phase is the numbness, his second phase yearning and protest, his third is disorganisation and despair, and lastly he describes the phase where recovery commences. The numbness that Parkes (1999) describes in phase one is accompanied by a feeling that it is all unreal, the bereaved cannot quite believe what has happened. This may last for a few hours or a few days. Yearning and protest in phase two are manifested by a tendency to cry, alternating with periods of anxiety and tension. The bereaved may display anger or bewilderment; this anxiety may escalate into panic attacks. Phase three brings despair and apathy. Bereaved people may lose their appetite, not only for food but for life in general; they may be unable to look or think about a future, living merely from day to day. Gradually, their appetite returns as they enter phase four, where recovery commences. The bereaved may be able to think of holidays, and they are more motivated to socialise and interact again with their wider social circle.

However, there is no end-point to grief (Parkes 1999) and the bereaved may still occasionally experience symptoms, which were associated with the grief in the early days, many years after the bereavement. Parkes, in his study of London widows (1971), found that he was able to establish a pattern of normal grief, and that certain factors (determinants of grief) affected the grieving process.

Determinants of grief

The identification of risk factors has implications for bereavement recovery. Different studies have found a number of factors that can be utilised to predict the outcome of bereavement on an individual. Parkes (1998) described the risk factors as: the place of death, successive deaths, the nature of the death, social network, attachment and loss history, age, and the complexity of the relationship with the deceased. Worden (1991) asks who the deceased was (spouse, child, parent), what was the nature of the attachment (was it a dependent or ambivalent relationship), the mode of death, the personality of the bereaved, and also about previous losses, social variables and other stresses present. The list identified by Bowlby (1981) included the identity and role of the deceased, the sex and personality of the bereaved and the circumstances of the death. Other factors, identified by various authors, include the bereaved person's history of previous losses, especially childhood loss or multiple losses. Previous mental health problems may also have an impact, or if there have been problems grieving in the past (Brennan 2004).

However, the experience of bereavement is considerably influenced not only by the above, but also by the wider society in which bereaved individuals live. Their cultural heritage, their beliefs, their family circumstances and perceived social support are also important factors that may influence the bereavement recovery. For example, what are the gender rules regarding an open display of grief, what beliefs are held about the future of the dead person, what are the prescribed cultural or religious rituals regarding death and bereavement and is the death stigmatised within the person's culture (Richards and Hare 1995)? Although these factors cannot necessarily predict an individual's reaction to grief, they can be used as a guide by the health care professionals, and especially the community palliative care clinical nurse specialist, in the assessment of the individual and also in providing the ongoing bereavement support to the bereaved carer or family.

Circumstances surrounding the death

Grief reactions may be determined to some extent by the circumstances surrounding the death. Even with cancer and other life-threatening illnesses, the patient may have a sudden or unexpected death. The illness trajectory may have been very short, or the patient may have deteriorated very quickly and died sooner than had been anticipated. In these circumstances the bereaved have little time to prepare for the death of their loved one and the loss is particularly devastating. There may have been no opportunity to say a last good-bye and indeed the carer may not have been present at the time of death; for some this will be especially difficult and result in feelings of guilt. Mental health problems such as anxiety, depression and post traumatic stress disorder may present in the bereaved after a sudden or unexpected death (Steen 1998). In certain circumstances, the death may be particularly traumatic, such as in a sudden catastrophic haemorrhage. If this is witnessed by the carer or family, they will need the opportunity, over the following weeks and months, to recount the event and express their distressing emotions. They may need considerable bereavement support from a variety of health professionals.

Case Story: Duncan

Duncan had lung cancer and lived with his wife. One morning she left Duncan in bed whilst she went to prepare the breakfast. After a few minutes she was aware of a noise and went to investigate. Duncan fell in front of her in the living room, there was blood pouring from his mouth and nose. He lost consciousness very quickly and died before she had time to call an ambulance. There was a trail of blood from the bedroom, into the bathroom, along the hall and into the living-room. The blood was everywhere, on the bed linen, on door handles, spatters on the walls and furniture and a large stain on the carpet; the house resembled a vicious crime scene. His wife could not stay in the house and their daughter arranged for her to stay with family whilst the house was professionally cleaned. Duncan's wife had known about the possibility of a haemorrhage, but she reported that nothing could have prepared her for the actual event. She not only required support from the community palliative care clinical nurse specialist, but also was referred on to professional bereavement counselling. Her nightmares and fearful emotions persisted for many, many months.

Although death from a massive haemorrhage is not a common occurrence, the health professional has to be aware of the possibility of a bleed in some patients and try to prepare individuals and their carers for this traumatic event. As illustrated from the above scenario, it is never possible to fully prepare anyone for what may happen. The community palliative care clinical nurse specialist, when giving information about possible life-threatening events, also has to take into account the amount of anxiety this information may create, and therefore it may be difficult to achieve a balance between preparing the carer in advance and causing more stress and worry about a situation that may or may not arise. However, research has shown that sudden, unexpected deaths can predispose to mental health problems in the bereaved, even when no other risk factors are present (Parkes 1998). It is therefore essential for risk assessments to be carried out by the health care professional, both pre and post bereavement, to determine the factors that may contribute to a complicated grief reaction.

In general, those who are prepared for a death are likely to do better in bereavement than those who experience a sudden or unexpected death (Monroe and Sheldon 2004). However, it has to be noted that a very long, protracted death can also result in bereavement problems (Doyle and Jeffrey 2000). This is also true when the survivor may have centred his or her life on caring for the sick loved one for many months or years (Parkes 1999).

The community palliative care clinical nurse specialist can therefore play a part in preparing families for the death of their loved one, by allowing emotions and fears to be expressed, giving support and advice, providing them with information and assessing the risk factors. Good palliative care involves planning and anticipating potential risks and offering supportive care; ideally the bereavement care should start before the death of the patient (Barry and Prigerson 2002). This requires the family and carer to be given as much information about the impending death as they desire, and also to inform them about bereavement and the anticipated reactions to grief. The community palliative care clinical nurse specialist can give time to carers to allow them the opportunity to express their emotions and prepare them for the death. This element of time may be unique to the community palliative care clinical nurse specialist compared to the other members of the health care team, who may be too busy to sit and allow grieving family to divulge their feelings. The community palliative care clinical nurse specialist can assess the carers and ascertain risk factors whilst listening to their anxieties. Help and support aimed at those individuals most at risk has been shown to be effective in improving outcome.

Age as a determinant of risk

Studies demonstrate that age appears to be a contributing factor when discussing determinants affecting grief outcome; although the literature can be conflicting in this respect. After the death of a partner, younger women are reported to be more at risk of poor bereavement outcome than their older counterparts (Steen 1998; Doyle and Jeffrey 2000; Woof and Nyatanga 2004). However, it has been found that older widows tend to consult their general practitioners with more physical complaints after bereavement, whilst the younger widows will look for emotional support (Monroe and Sheldon 2004).

This may be a generational anomaly as today's older population have traditionally been less inclined to articulate their emotions to others, whilst the younger generations are more adept at expressing themselves and seeking help with their feelings. If the age of the deceased is taken into consideration, there is undoubtedly a difference in today's society between the expected death of an elderly individual and the untimely death of a younger person. However, the elderly may have many other losses to tolerate at the same time as their bereavement, such as loss of their own health, loss of their independence and perhaps loss of their home due to their failing health and inability to care for themselves after their partner dies. Indeed Parkes (1998) reports that there is evidence that older individuals are more susceptible to the effects of bereavement on their physical health and this is bound to have ongoing consequences.

This has implications for the community palliative care clinical nurse specialist who then needs to not only prepare individuals for the loss of their loved one, but also anticipate and plan the care for the bereaved after the death. Support is therefore just as important for the bereaved elderly as it is for younger individuals; however, it may be of a different nature depending on their needs.

Case Story: Pamela

Pamela (81) had suffered a stroke many years ago and had been dependent on her husband for assistance around the home and with shopping, etc. She could manage to attend her own personal hygiene needs, but her mobility was severely limited. Her husband had bowel cancer and was now very unwell. Maximum assistance had been organised for the couple, but it was becoming increasingly difficult for them to cope at home. The community palliative care clinical nurse specialist had known the couple for some time and had to broach the difficult subject of ongoing care for Pamela and her husband. It was agreed that Pamela would have to move into a nursing home after her husband's death; however, they wanted to try to allow her husband to die at home. They both felt that it would be easier for Pamela to leave the family home after her husband's death, rather than coping with another loss at present. The couple used their savings to purchase 24-hour private nursing care at home, achieving her husband's wish to die in his own bed. The community palliative care clinical nurse specialist visited Pamela in the nursing home to give ongoing bereavement support. Pamela had not only the loss of her husband to endure, but also the loss of her own health, her independence and the loss of her home.

The community palliative care clinical nurse specialist will offer support to the carers and families of all the patients with whom she has had contact. This is irrespective of their age, their risk assessment or the circumstances surrounding the death. It should be noted, however, that the author is describing her own role in bereavement support and is very aware that there are variations in the way community palliative care clinical nurse specialists will function, and the support offered will depend on the role of each particular nurse and her employing authority. Many areas have local bereavement services available and referrals may be passed on to the bereavement coordinator, with only minimal contact from the community palliative care clinical nurse specialist after the patient's death. Nevertheless, all community palliative care clinical nurse specialists will have the knowledge and skills to assess the bereaved and support appropriately.

Relationships and personalities

The community palliative care clinical nurse specialist will be aware that the relationship between the bereaved and the deceased is also a determinant factor in explaining the response to the death. For example, the loss of a husband or partner will usually give rise to more psychological difficulties than the death of an elderly parent. A grandparent, who dies at an elderly age, will be grieved differently than a sibling whose premature death resulted from cancer or other life-threatening illness. The nature of the attachment between the deceased and the bereaved may also influence the grieving process. Marital relationships can be complex and may influence the health and well-being of the bereaved survivor (Ott et al. 2007). Personal relationships are not always as they appear to outsiders, or to the health care professionals. Some relationships are dependent, abusive, ambivalent or complex in other ways. Individuals with a particularly ambivalent relationship have an increased likelihood of a difficult grief reaction (Doyle and Jeffrey 2000) and may experience an immense amount of guilt and anger (Worden 1991). The bereaved may feel that he/she has been deprived of the opportunity to resolve unfinished emotional issues with the deceased. However, not all deaths will be regarded by the bereaved as a trauma, nor will they present with grief-related problems. For some individuals the death may result in a new sense of freedom and a new life.

Case Story: Muriel

Muriel was an unmarried lady of 56 years of age. She had cared for her elderly parents for many years. Her mother had died of dementia some years before and her father had recently died of bowel cancer. Muriel declined any ongoing bereavement support from the community palliative care clinical nurse specialist. She reported that her parents had been elderly; she had been well prepared for their deaths and knew she had cared for them to the best of her abilities, allowing both to die at home. She now wanted to rejoin the many groups and activities that she had given up over the years and visit friends overseas. She felt that she could now move on with her own life after many years of being a carer.

The personality of the bereaved has also to be taken into account when trying to understand an individual's response to loss (Worden 1991).

In the above scenario, the bereaved individual had coped well with the stress of caring for her parents and had been well prepared for their deaths. Others may have poor coping abilities and manifest a high degree of anxiety prior to and after the death of their loved one. Bereavement is also associated with increased health-threatening behaviours such as smoking, drinking and drug use (Twycross 1999). Reactions to bereavement will also depend on the individual's previous losses, particularly other significant deaths. The ability of the health care professionals to predict the course of grief will never be perfect, as there are too many variables which may intervene; however, the role of the community palliative care clinical nurse specialist incorporates a proactive approach in assessing bereaved individuals and offering support and intervention where needed.

Normal/abnormal grief

Normal grief, sometimes referred to as uncomplicated grief, incorporates a wide range of emotions and behaviours that are experienced after a loss. Grief is a painful process, with many strong emotions, and is experienced, to a lesser or greater extent, by those individuals affected by the death of a loved one. Grief may be lonely, soul-destroying, difficult and depressing (Neuberger 2004). The grief may vary in intensity and in the length of time to individual recovery. The grieving process usually starts before the death and may be as early as when the patient is informed that his or her illness is incurable. Both the patient and carer will feel the impending loss and it is not uncommon for the patient and family to grieve together (Palmer and Howarth 2005).

This anticipatory grief may be difficult to express because of the carers' need to protect the patient and vice versa. Carers may want to keep a degree of control on their emotions, fearing that they may be unable to cope with the enormity of the situation if they allow themselves to become upset. This at times is a defence mechanism and a way of handling their distressing situation; it would be wrong of the health care professional to assert undue pressure on carers and dismantle their way of coping (Parkes 1999). However, over a period of time, this will be difficult to maintain and the carer will need the support of a professional, such as the community palliative care clinical nurse specialist, to intervene and offer supportive care.

Anticipatory grief sees the family trying to imagine what life will be like without their loved one, trying to mentally adjust to the future, and will most certainly be accompanied by fears of abandonment, helplessness and anxiety (Grassi 2007). This can be a difficult time for the family or carers, as the patient's illness trajectory may be punctuated by periods of relatively good health, and they may find that the rollercoaster of emotions they experience leaves them exhausted and confused. At times, the patient and carer may not be able to discuss their complex emotions with one another, usually for fear of upsetting the other party, and their feelings of grief may deepen as a result of the conspiracy of silence (Doyle and Jeffrey 2000).

At times, particularly after a lingering illness, considerable grieving has been done by the time the patient dies; this may leave the survivor with a feeling of relief, rather than grief (Palmer and Howarth 2005) and, as a result, individuals may feel surprised by or guilty with their emotions. In general, the health care team members who have cared for the deceased during the illness should ensure that the bereaved have adequate emotional support after the death (Brennan 2004). For many, their world now seems empty and their lives have no purpose, their future may seem futile and full of uncertainty. Undertaking a risk assessment will help to determine what support the bereaved may have in their community and also their perceived support. This will allow the health care team to determine which individuals will benefit from supportive intervention. Care needs to be taken, however, in emphasising that grief is a normal response to loss and that it should not be medicalised. Most individuals have adequate coping abilities to work through their grief, and interference in that process by outsiders or professionals may lead to a disempowerment of the bereaved and be detrimental in their return to normal life.

Knowledge of the theories surrounding grief and the emotions and behaviours that individuals experience (discussed earlier in this chapter) is essential for the health care professionals to assist the bereaved in their journey. Normal grief is an understanding of the effects of bereavement upon individuals in general and can be described in terms of stages or tasks. However, one of the difficulties in this approach is that people do not pass through the stages in a strict order; instead the stages tend to overlap. Individuals may seem to miss one stage, move backwards or forwards or get stuck in a particular stage (Palmer and Howarth 2005). The vast majority of bereaved are able to work through these stages or phases on their own and need minimal or no intervention from professionals.

Essentially, the bereaved individual has to adjust to a world where the deceased is no longer present (Brennan 2004). Normal grieving is a self-limiting process that, despite the many strong emotions which may accompany its course, does resolve and individuals do achieve recovery (Doyle and Jeffrey 2000). However, although grief is a normal response to the death of a loved one, families may still need help with their problems and emotions. Talking about their grief can be therapeutic and may be all that is required for many people (Brennan 2004). Some bereaved individuals may appreciate support from the community palliative care clinical nurse specialist to work through the normal stages of grief, and, with help and encouragement, through time, they can again resume a more normal life. However, a small number of people will discover that they have difficulty with their feelings and are unable to complete their recovery and return to normal life. These individuals may develop significant problems relating to their loss and may benefit from skilled therapeutic intervention (Palmer and Howarth 2005).

Abnormal or complicated grief

Individuals vary enormously in their experience of grief, and therefore assessing whether grief is normal or abnormal is complex (Thomas 2003). Some people fail to grieve in the normal way or take longer than average to reach a particular phase. However, it is unhelpful to be prescriptive regarding the normal course of grief, because there are so many variables determined by personal and cultural influences. Identifying the differing patterns of grief, however, is of clinical relevance in determining those most likely to benefit from supportive intervention (Ott et al. 2007). The community palliative care clinical nurse specialist needs to be aware of the difficulties some individuals may face and be familiar with, and able to identify, the main forms of complicated grief. For some individuals, features of normal grieving overlap those of depression, post-traumatic stress disorder, substance abuse and bereavement disorders (Doyle and Jeffrey 2000). Individuals with complicated grief reactions will inevitably require referral on to other appropriate agencies for therapeutic intervention.

Chronic grief

A chronic grief reaction is one that is excessive in duration, where the person is unable to return to normal living (Worden 1991; Lugton and Kindlen 1999; Doyle and Jeffrey 2000; Brennan 2004). According to Doyle and Jeffrey (2000), this most often occurs in highly dependent relationships, whilst Palmer and Howarth (2005) suggest it can be seen in individuals with an emotional or dramatic personality. Irrespective of the personality, the individual becomes stuck and unable to move forwards, either in goal setting or forming new relationships. They appear to withdraw into their grief and may still be mourning many years later. This type of grief reaction is quite easy to determine, as the bereaved are usually aware that they are not progressing and the grief is unfinished (Worden 1991).

Delayed grief

In this situation, the bereaved individual may have had an initial reaction to the loss, but then appears to recover very quickly and carries on as usual. The reason for the delayed grief may be that the bereaved is overburdened at the time of the original loss and unable to express emotions; such as in the case of a lone parent or the family breadwinner. They may also be overwhelmed by more than one loss or a highly stressful event, leading them to put their own grief aside, to try to resolve these other issues (Brennan 2004). However, the reaction is only delayed until a point in the future when emotions return with great intensity (Lugton and Kindlen 1999). The trigger that acts as a catalyst for the future response may be another loss or even an emotional situation such as a sad movie and may at the time be quite insignificant in nature. This may, however, precipitate a powerful and excessive grief reaction and the individual will be aware that it is out of proportion to the current situation. What happens is that some of the grieving that was not adequately completed at the time of the original loss is carried forward and experienced at the time of the subsequent loss or emotional situation (Worden 1991).

Masked grief

Masked grief arises when a delayed grief reaction manifests itself as some other problem. The person may be experiencing physical symptoms (similar to those of the deceased) or psychological problems such as depression or a phobia and these can mask an underlying loss that has not been fully resolved (Brennan 2004). The bereaved experience these problems, but do not recognise the fact that they are related to their bereavement (Worden 1991).

Exaggerated grief

This can occur when the bereaved individual becomes completely engulfed in their emotions and may develop severe depression or become dependent on alcohol or drugs (Lugton and Kindlen 1999). People experiencing exaggerated grief are aware that the difficulties they are encountering are connected to their loss and may seek help. Their problems may at times be excessive and disabling, and may manifest as major psychiatric disorders (Worden 1991).

The categories of abnormal grief described often appear as mixed scenarios, but clearly the greater the number of risk factors, the greater the risk of abnormal grief. The results of a study by Ott et al. (2007) describe an emerging trend toward the use of the terms common grief, resiliency in grief and chronic grief; however, the main issue is that the community palliative care clinical nurse specialist is able to identify how individuals are coping with their grief and take relevant steps for intervention when necessary. Where abnormal grief is identified, referral to clinical psychology or psychiatric services may be appropriate. However, many of the problems and pathology associated with abnormal bereavement can be avoided by work before the death, endeavouring to minimise the effect of factors that increase the risk of poor outcome.

The community palliative care clinical nurse specialist is ideally placed to support the carers prior to the death, to carry out an assessment to determine the possible risk factors for poor bereavement outcome and to offer ongoing support into the bereavement period.

Bereavement trajectories

Parkes (1998) believes that the reluctance to change, to give up people, possessions, status and expectations is the basis to grief. His concept of psychosocial transitions has suggested that certain events, such as bereavement, lead to major changes in the individual's life, and in grief the individual has to develop a new set of assumptions about his or her world. Parkes (1971) describes four phases of grieving, although reports that the transitions from one phase to another are seldom distinct. In order to further demonstrate the response that individuals may have after bereavement, the ensuing case histories will describe the grief reactions of two widows. They will describe their bereavement trajectories in relation to the Parkes model and the support and intervention given by the community palliative care clinical nurse specialist.

Family history – profile 1

Elizabeth is a 50-year-old mother of five teenage children. She works in a large retail outlet. The family moved into the area 4 years ago in response to an improved employment opportunity for her husband. Her own family live some distance away, but are supportive and visit whenever possible. Elizabeth's husband Bobby died last year from a haematological cancer. He was 53 years of age and had been diagnosed with cancer 2 years previously. His illness had necessitated lengthy stays in hospital, and towards the end of his life he had been an inpatient for several months in a large cancer unit some distance from home. When Elizabeth was informed that Bobby was dying, she requested that he be transferred to the small local hospice. He died 2 weeks later, with his family at his bedside.

Elizabeth's husband had been in hospital for lengthy periods during the last years of his life. She had had to change and adapt to her new role in managing the family affairs and looking after their busy teenage children. Bobby and Elizabeth had discussed her future and made all the arrangements to simplify life for the family after his death. She had always found the hospital staff helpful and her own general practitioner had given time to listen to Elizabeth on the occasions when she visited him. Elizabeth had had the opportunity to express her worries and fears prior to and after Bobby's death with a 'befriender' (a trained volunteer) at the hospice. Several days after Bobby's death, the general practitioner asked the community palliative care clinical nurse specialist to visit Elizabeth, to assess and assist with the grieving process.

Phase one

Parkes (1971) states that the first phase of grief is numbness and that it can start within minutes of the death and last from a few hours to a few days. Elizabeth reported that this period of numbness and shock allowed her time to arrange the funeral. According to Stroebe et al. (1993), the gathering of relatives for the funeral can facilitate passage through this phase. Elizabeth reported the funeral helpful as it gave a sense of reality to the situation.

Phase two

The second phase has two independent components: yearning and protest (Parkes 1971). The initial numbness gives way to a period of strong emotions as the awareness of the loss develops. Intense yearning accompanies this and is characterised by pangs of grief, which are thought to be the principal feature of the urge to reunite with the loved one (Parkes 1971). Elizabeth experienced strong feelings and described these as similar to 'panic attacks'. Feelings of panic and other indications of autonomic activity are particularly pronounced during pangs of grief (Parkes 1998). Elizabeth reported the attacks as disturbing, but gradually their frequency and severity subsided.

Stroebe and Stroebe (1987) describe a feature of this phase as searching for the deceased. Elizabeth found her need to be reunited with her husband very strong. She found difficulty in sleeping and interpreted noises in the night as Bobby trying to communicate with her and this precipitated a visit to a spiritualist. Parkes (1998) reports that spiritualism claims to help individuals in their search for the dead. However, his study of London widows (1971) revealed that individuals did not feel satisfied by the experience. Indeed, Elizabeth felt frightened by her visit and declined to return.

From his London study (1971), Parkes noted that irritability and anger feature in the second phase. Elizabeth expressed irritability with the children, shouting at them and directing her anger towards them. As a result the children stayed out more with their friends. Elizabeth's brother was very supportive at this time, staying with his sister and also speaking to the children about their feelings. As the second phase progresses, the tearfulness and anxiety are the first features to decline, with the irritability decreasing more gradually throughout the first year (Parkes 1971). However, it is stated that there is no end-point to yearning, and pangs of grief can be felt years after the bereavement. As yearning diminishes there seems to follow a period of uncertainty and apathy, which is called disorganisation and despair (Parkes 1998).

Phase three

Elizabeth became withdrawn and declined to discuss her future. Her general practitioner prescribed anti-depressants, but Elizabeth refused to take them and also admitted to drinking more alcohol than was her normal consumption. Parkes (1998) states that the efficacy of anti-depressants in normal grief has not been demonstrated and that dependence on alcohol is a real danger after bereavement. The process of overcoming apathy and depression is slow (Stroebe and Stroebe 1987), and only when circumstances force her will the widow venture out and reintegrate into society (Parkes 1998). As Christmas was now approaching, Elizabeth felt that she had to make an effort for her children. Parkes (1998) states that a mother may find that the care of the children provides her with a purpose in her life. Four months had passed since Bobby's death and Elizabeth had started working again and was now able to deal with Bobby's clothing and personal belongings. For most individuals the episodes of depression and hopelessness begin to be mixed with more positive feelings (Stroebe and Stroebe 1987).

Phase four

This phase sees the reorganised behaviour when the bereaved begins to invest in life again. As the months passed, Elizabeth became more confident in her new role and her altered social status; her relationship with her children strengthened and they planned to have a family holiday just before the anniversary of Bobby's death. Parkes (1998) states that it takes time for individuals to realise and accept the change in themselves that follows a major loss. However, in the normal course of events, the widowed will appreciate that life without the partner is feasible and that coping alone is possible.

Family history – profile 2

Cheryl is a 24-year-old who lives near to her parents. Cheryl had been 'going steady' with Jack since she was 14 years of age; she finds it difficult to remember a time when he was not part of her life. Cheryl and Jack had been married for just over a year and had been hoping to start a family soon. Cheryl's family and friends visited often and the house was usually very busy. Jack found a lump on his shoulder 18 months ago; he was 25 years old. With persuasion from Cheryl, he visited the doctor. It was removed and found to be a malignant melanoma. Cheryl and Jack did not realise the possible consequences of this diagnosis and Jack missed several follow-up appointments. When the general practitioner urged Jack to attend for review many months later, the cancer was discovered to have metastasised. Unfortunately Jack's condition deteriorated very rapidly and he died only 2 days after Cheryl recognised he was dying.

Cheryl expressed anger towards the doctors at the hospital. She had spoken to them only once about Jack's condition, but had not understood what had been said at the time. The general practitioner only became aware of the rapid deterioration in Jack's condition a few days before his death and encouraged Cheryl to allow the community palliative care clinical nurse specialist to visit; she very reluctantly agreed. The community palliative care clinical nurse specialist visited 2 days before Jack died; this was the first time Cheryl talked about the possibility of Jack dying. His death, 48 hours later, was a catastrophic event in Cheryl's life.

Phase one

Stroebe and Stroebe (1987) report that, for most widows, grief runs a normal course; for others the effects are devastating. Wright (1996) reports that many bereaved people are concerned at their immediate numbness and lack of feeling. Cheryl not only experienced numbness, but also reported disbelief. She voiced concerns that she was *empty* and uncomfortable with her lack of emotions. According to Kendrick (1998), a sense of disbelief and unreality are common initial responses. Cheryl found no comfort in the funeral; she had been unable to cry.

Four weeks after Jack's death, Cheryl was still feeling numb. Stroebe et al. (2003) report that one of the difficulties for those who are bereaved is that there is no clear format of how they should feel. They state that some individuals display no post-death emotions. The absence of these emotions can be conscious (such as delayed grief due to the necessity of dealing with issues such as family or finance) or unconscious (such as the bereaved not believing the loved one is dead). Cheryl was concerned about her feelings and frequently contacted the community palliative care clinical nurse specialist for advice and reassurance. She also referred herself to a CRUSE bereavement counsellor (CRUSE is an organisation, established in 1958, that provides a range of services to the bereaved, including counselling by trained counsellors).

According to Parkes (1998), the first source of help for most bereaved should be their family. Cheryl's family were supportive and her sister stayed with Cheryl overnight for many weeks. However, Jack's parents had difficulty coping with the loss of their only son and found it very painful trying to give support to Cheryl. Her parents thought that a break away to her grandparents might be of benefit to their daughter.

Cheryl felt uncomfortable when she was away and on returning home was confronted by the emptiness of the house; suddenly she started to cry. Cheryl realised that Jack was not going to return. Cheryl had experienced numbness for 9 weeks.

Phase two

The second phase, described as 'acute mourning' by Stroebe et al. (1993), begins when the death has been acknowledged both cognitively and emotionally. Cheryl now experienced pangs of grief and feelings of panic overcame Cheryl both day and night; they would leave her sobbing and distraught. She was restless and tried to keep herself busy by continually producing lists of things needing attention. Parkes (1971) affirms that hyperactivity is a feature of the reaction to bereavement. Cheryl's emotions turned to anger. Raphael (1986) states that the bereaved are angry because they feel deserted by the deceased. Cheryl's anger was directed at the professionals who had been involved in her husband's care. Anger can often be aimed at those whose actions were thought to have harmed the loved one prior to death. Cheryl was also experiencing extreme guilt because she had not encouraged Jack to seek advice earlier and had allowed the follow-up appointments to be cancelled. She felt that she was in some way to blame for Jack's death. Penson (1990) reports that with an illness such as cancer, many people express guilt for not interpreting the early signs of the disease as being potentially dangerous.

Cheryl found sleep difficult and had visions in which she saw Jack in his coffin. Parkes (1998) states that hallucinations can be interpreted as a sign of insanity and therefore it can be alarming to experience the hypnagogic hallucinations of a dead husband. Hallucinatory experiences are indeed commonplace and most manifest in the form of *sensing* the presence of the dead spouse. Noises at night disturbed Cheryl; she felt Jack's presence in the house and was uncomfortable with these feelings. However, as time passes the intensity and frequency of the strong emotions diminish and then the period of apathy and despair begins.

Phase three

Cheryl lost interest in her lists. Over 7 months had passed since Jack had died and she continued to have difficulties sleeping at night.

Cheryl's general practitioner was concerned that she was becoming clinically depressed, but refrained from the use of anti-depressants and continued to monitor the situation. According to Ott et al. (2007), depressive symptoms tend to diminish over time and do not indicate a need for professional intervention. Cheryl was continuing to have regular counselling from CRUSE bereavement services and the community palliative care clinical nurse specialist was visiting the house frequently. Cheryl's mother now felt that Cheryl should be coping with the loss in a more positive way and started spending less time with her daughter. Cheryl's sister, who had been staying overnight for several months, also wanted to move back to her own family and gradually reduced the number of nights per week she stayed at Cheryl's house. Cheryl was upset by this and felt her family should be more supportive. The reality was that her sister's husband was beginning to get upset at his wife's continued absence from their home and Cheryl's mother was emotionally exhausted trying to support her daughter. Cheryl subsequently turned to friends and asked them to stay each night. This proved difficult to sustain and gradually Cheryl had to endure nights alone. This was very difficult initially, but over the following months Cheryl managed to adjust to being alone in the house and began to slowly realise that she had developed new skills in maintaining the house and garden. This gave her back some confidence and 9 months after Jack's death she managed to return to her work as a class-room assistant.

Phase four

For many widows it takes a considerable period of time to realise what it is like to live without their husbands (Worden 1991). Cheryl gradually adapted to life without Jack and even managed to sort out his clothes and possessions shortly before the first anniversary of his death. She began to socialise again and started talking about a more positive future. The input from the community palliative care clinical nurse specialist gradually reduced from regular visits to telephone contact and eventually Cheryl reported that she would phone if needed. She also stopped the CRUSE bereavement counselling not long after the first anniversary, reporting that there were others who 'would need them'. Bowlby (1981) reports that most women take a long time to get over the death of a husband and less than half are *themselves* again at the end of the first year.

Support systems

Bereavement support requires a range of skills, with communication playing a vital role. The main tasks are to provide an environment where the bereaved feel able to talk, to reassure them of the normality of the emotions and help direct them towards realistic adjustment to their new pattern of life (Penson 1990). It is important for those who help the bereaved to know what is normal and also to feel comfortable in supporting them. The community palliative care clinical nurse specialist has the knowledge and skills to facilitate the bereaved in their journey. Indeed, many community palliative care clinical nurse specialists may have undertaken not only counselling courses, but also further training in bereavement counselling. It is also particularly important for professionals to appreciate that their role is one of facilitator rather than that of problem solver (Faulkner 1998).

Elizabeth had been well supported prior to Bobby's death and found the hospital staff to be honest and informative when discussing issues about Bobby's illness. She also found comfort from her contacts with the general practitioner and the volunteer befriender had been very supportive. After Bobby's death, the community palliative care clinical nurse specialist had been asked to provide support. Parkes (1999) states that a stranger coming in for the first time after a death may be seen as an intruder, whereas someone already known to the family is more acceptable. Therefore it might be argued that the community palliative care clinical nurse specialist was not the most appropriate professional to provide ongoing bereavement support to Elizabeth. However, Elizabeth had now severed contact with the hospital and did not feel that she wanted to return to the hospice for bereavement support; she was in agreement when the general practitioner suggested that the community palliative care clinical nurse specialist would provide the necessary support after Bobby's death.

Bereavement support may involve direct visitation, telephone contact or formal bereavement counselling. The community palliative care clinical nurse specialist initially made telephone contact with Elizabeth and arranged to meet her at home. The purpose of a bereavement visit is to assess whether grieving has commenced, if grief is within normal limits and whether there is any sign that adaptation has started (Faulkner 1998). During the visits, Elizabeth expressed her feelings, actualised the loss by talking about Bobby's death and discussed effective coping and decision-making skills. Continued support is necessary for some bereaved individuals and may be needed for many months. Visits continued until Elizabeth resumed work and then telephone contact allowed Elizabeth to keep in touch if needed. Elizabeth felt she had a supportive network of family and friends who helped when needed and listened when she wanted to talk about her feelings. The community palliative care clinical nurse specialist was confident that Elizabeth's grief was normal and allowed this supportive network to continue to be Elizabeth's mainstay of support.

Cheryl had found the period prior to Jack's death difficult, partly due to her perceived lack of information. Her first contact with any community support, instigated by the general practitioner, was just 48 hours before Jack's death. The initial visit by the community palliative care clinical nurse specialist revealed that Cheryl had been uncomfortable discussing issues with the hospital doctors. However, given time and the secure surroundings of her own home, she was able to express her feelings and concerns, assimilate the information she had been given and start to understand the reality of the situation.

Parkes (1998) states that for most people in the early stages of bereavement the world is in chaos; however, Cheryl was very organised initially and talked about her plans for the house. She showed no sadness or tears during the early visits. The community palliative care clinical nurse specialist was concerned about Cheryl's reactions and, fearing a potentially abnormal grief response, visited more regularly to assist Cheryl to work through her grief. It has been discussed earlier in this chapter that under-reaction to grief requires attention, as delayed responses may be destructive later. Indeed the community palliative care clinical nurse specialist invested many hours in visits to Cheryl, but this did eventually prove to be effective when small improvements were noted in Cheryl's grieving. Very gradually, Cheryl began to express her feelings, her loneliness and the enormity of Jack's death in her life. Several months after Jack's death, the health care professionals were still expressing some concerns about Cheryl's grieving and also her mental health; however, she did demonstrate some indication of progress through the stages of grief, even if it was very slowly. Cheryl had been forced to spend time alone in the house, but this had helped her to gain new skills. The more successful the bereaved are in achieving new roles and skills, the more confident and independent they begin to feel (Bowlby 1981). The community palliative care clinical nurse specialist continued to visit until Cheryl felt confident to discontinue the direct contact. Parkes (1999) reports that grief lasts a long time; however, there is no need to expect that professional support should continue until the bereaved have come through their grief, but it is important to ensure that they are on course to attain recovery.

The time scale of grief reactions varies considerably and may be helped or hindered by the support available. There is no doubt, however, that the support and information given before the death will reduce the risk of poor bereavement outcomes. According to Parkes (1998), those who are concerned with bereavement have to take into consideration many possible determinants when explaining the differences between individuals and responses. There is no shortage of claims for attaching importance to age, sex, personality and other factors, but the findings are far from consistent and each person who has studied bereavement seems to have produced a different list (Parkes and Weiss 1983).

Parkes (1998) reports that the widows studied were clearly more emotionally disturbed following deaths for which they had little time to prepare. He states that unexpected deaths were found to give rise to a characteristic type of response; the initial reactions of numbness and disbelief persisted for a considerable time and were associated with a continuing sense of the presence of the dead person. The community palliative care clinical nurse specialist has to be aware of these reactions when visiting the bereaved and intervene appropriately to give support. In the above family histories, Cheryl was unprepared for her husband's death and had a difficult grief reaction, whilst Elizabeth had been given information and had time and the opportunity to prepare for her loved one's death. Both widows, however, with time and support from the community palliative care clinical nurse specialist and others, managed to work through the phases of grief and regain some semblance of normal living without their husbands.

Social network

An important factor in the way that individuals cope with their grief is the support they receive within their family and social network (Faulkner 1998). The family and the social network surrounding the bereaved person are one of the key factors protecting them from the detrimental effects of loss. However, in today's society the bereaved may be unable to rely on their family and friends to stand by and help them in their distress; this has resulted in increasing reliance upon professionals and volunteer counsellors to give the necessary help to the bereaved.

From the family histories, it was demonstrated that Elizabeth felt well supported by her family and friends. However, due to their lack of understanding of the grief process, Cheryl's family and friends allowed their support to wane before Cheryl was ready to cope on her own. She had found the lack of support from Jack's parents particularly distressing. It has been reported, however, that many widows claim that their husband's family loses all interest in them after the death (Raphael 1985). For many, the support of the professionals does not compensate for the perceived loss of support from family and friends. Although the relationship between risk factors and outcome is complex, if individuals are given the opportunity to grieve, they should eventually progress to feeling confident and positive about their future life.

Offering support

The community palliative care clinical nurse specialist is a member of the wider primary health care team and as such will liaise, communicate and participate in the care of patients and their families alongside fellow colleagues. Individual members of the team will offer support to the patient and carers prior to the patient's death; however, their continued support may not extend into the bereavement period beyond a single post-death visit. The role of the community palliative care clinical nurse specialist, as explained previously, extends beyond the immediate post-death visit to offer support for many months if required.

Grief and bereavement should be viewed as a continuum, with assessment and support of the carer and family ideally commencing before the death of their loved one (Grassi 2007). The assessment of risk factors should therefore be carried out prior to the death of the patient, and those family members most likely to be significantly affected by the death should be targeted. The risk assessment may be undertaken by any member of the primary health care team, but, in reality, it may well be the community palliative care clinical nurse specialist who performs this assessment. This may partly result from her anticipated continuing intervention post death with the bereaved family members. It should be remembered, however, that limited resources may be a disadvantage in offering ongoing support to all bereaved, and therefore a more efficient and effective service will be achieved, with greater benefit to bereaved individuals, if those most likely to be at risk are targeted. The use of a bereavement risk assessment tool or bereavement scale will provide a consistent and recognised means of assessing the bereaved. There are many cited in the nursing literature; however, their explanation is beyond the scope of this text. What is important is that the tool chosen should be reliable and consistent, easy to use and that the professionals using the tool have been adequately trained in its usage.

The community palliative care clinical nurse specialist has to be aware of the physical as well as the emotional challenges faced by those individuals who have experienced the death of a loved one. The bereaved may suffer from anxiety, disturbed sleep patterns, poor appetite, various aches and pains, mood changes and difficulty in concentrating on tasks. The community palliative care clinical nurse specialist needs to address these issues and determine whether they are within the course of normal grief or whether they are abnormal. Many of these features are indeed experienced by the bereaved within the early part of their grief journey and are normal reactions to the bereavement. However, there is a reported increase in deaths from heart disease within the bereaved population, and figures also suggest significant incidences of depressive illness. It is therefore essential that those individuals who are at risk of poor bereavement outcome are identified and steps taken to offer supportive intervention to avert any significant pathology developing.

The community palliative care clinical nurse specialist has an important role to play in the support of the bereaved both prior to the death and after the death of the patient. An awareness of normal grief reactions and also abnormal grief will allow the community palliative care clinical nurse specialist to assess the bereaved and consider the relevant risks factors when determining the support required for the individuals. Many bereaved will appreciate an opportunity to talk about their emotions, but care has to be taken to ensure that the normal grief process is not medicalised and that they are allowed to continue through their journey, secure in the knowledge that supportive care is available from the community palliative care clinical nurse specialist if desired.

Key Points

- The death of a loved individual is an experience that everybody confronts at some point in life.
- The erosion of the extended family and the disregard of formal mourning have meant that the bereaved get little support from their families or society.

- One of the elements of palliative care is provision of support in bereavement; therefore the nursing care and responsibilities to the dying patient and their family do not end with the death of the patient (Matzo et al. 2003).
- The role of the community palliative care clinical nurse specialist includes facilitating the grief process by assessing grief, assisting the survivor to feel and express the loss and helping the bereaved to work through the stages of grief.
- Although most individuals possess adequate resources to cope with bereavement, for some the challenge can be difficult (Woof and Nyatanga 1998).
- The identification of risk factors has implications for bereavement recovery.
- Research has shown that sudden, unexpected deaths can predispose to mental health problems in the bereaved, even when no other risk factors are present (Parkes 1998).
- Studies demonstrate that age appears to be a contributing factor when discussing determinants affecting grief outcome, although the literature can be conflicting in this respect.
- The community palliative care clinical nurse specialist will be aware that the relationship between the bereaved and the deceased is also a determinant factor in explaining the response to the death.
- Normal grief, sometimes referred to as uncomplicated grief, incorporates a wide range of emotions and behaviours that are experienced after a loss.
- Individuals vary enormously in their experience of grief; therefore assessing whether grief is normal or abnormal is complex (Thomas 2003).
- Where abnormal grief is identified, referral to clinical psychology or psychiatric services may be appropriate.
- Bereavement support may involve direct visitation, telephone contact or formal bereavement counselling.
- Parkes (1999) reports that grief lasts a long time; however, there is no need to expect that professional support should continue until the bereaved have come through their grief, but it is important to ensure that they are on course to attain recovery.
- Grief and bereavement should be viewed as a continuum, with assessment and support of the carer and family ideally commencing before the death of their loved one (Grassi 2007).
- The community palliative care clinical nurse specialist has an important role to play in the support of the bereaved both prior to the death and after the death of the patient.

Useful resources

Brennan J (2004) *Cancer in Context: A Practical Guide to Supportive Care.* Oxford University Press, Oxford.

Grassi L (2007) Bereavement in families with relatives dying of cancer. *Current Opinion in Supportive and Palliative Care* 1 (1), 43–49.

Kubler-Ross E (1969) *On Death and Dying.* Macmillan, New York.

Lindemann E (1944) Symptomatology and management of acute grief. *American Journal of Psychiatry* 101, 141–148.

Neuberger J (2004) *Dying Well: A Guide to Enabling a Good Death,* 2nd edn. Radcliffe, Abingdon.

Ott C, Lueger RJ, Kelber ST, Prigerson HG (2007) Spousal bereavement in older adults: common, resilient and chronic grief with defining characteristics. *Journal of Nervous and Mental Disease* 195 (4), 332–341.

Parkes CM (1998) *Bereavement: Studies of Grief in Adult Life.* Penguin, London.

Stroebe MS, Stroebe W, Hanson RO (eds) (1993) *Handbook of Bereavement: Theory, Research and Intervention.* Cambridge University Press, Cambridge.

Worden JW (1991) *Grief Counselling and Grief Therapy: A Handbook for the Mental Health Practitioner,* 2nd edn. Routledge, London.

References

Barry LC, Prigerson HG (2002) Perspectives on preparedness for a death among bereaved persons. *Connecticut Medicine* 66 (11), 691–697.

Bowlby J (1981) *Attachment and Loss. Volume 3: Loss, Sadness and Depression.* Penguin, London.

Brennan J (2004) *Cancer in Context: A Practical Guide to Supportive Care.* Oxford University Press, Oxford.

Corr CA, Nabe CM, Corr DM (2003) *Death and Dying: Life and Living,* 4th edn. Wadsworth/Thomson Learning, Belmont.

Doyle D, Jeffrey D (2000) *Palliative Care in the Home.* Oxford University Press, Oxford.

Faulkner A (1998) *Working with Bereaved People.* Churchill Livingstone, Edinburgh.

Grassi L (2007) Bereavement in families with relatives dying of cancer. *Current Opinion in Supportive and Palliative Care* 1 (1), 43–49.

Kendrick K (1998) Bereavement part 1: theories of bereavement. *Professional Nurse* 14 (1), 59–62.

Kindlen M, Smith V, Smith M (1999) Loss grief and bereavement. In: Lugton J, Kindlen M (eds) *Palliative Care: The Nursing Role*, pp 217–248. Churchill Livingstone, Edinburgh.

Kubler-Ross E (1969) *On Death and Dying*. Macmillan, New York.

Lindemann E (1944) Symptomatology and management of acute grief. *American Journal of Psychiatry* 101, 141–148.

Main J (2002) Management of relatives who are dying. *Journal of Clinical Nursing* 11, 794–801.

Matzo ML, Sherman DW, Egan KA, Grant M, Rhome A (2003) Strategies for teaching loss, grief and bereavement. *Nurse Educator* 28 (2), 71–76.

Melliar-Smith C (2002) The risk assessment of bereavement in a palliative setting. *International Journal of Palliative Nursing* 8 (6), 281–287.

Monroe B, Sheldon F (2004) Psychosocial dimensions of care. In: Sykes N, Edmonds P, Wiles J (eds) *Management of Advanced Disease*, 4th edn, pp 405–437. Arnold, London.

Neuberger J (2004) *Dying Well: A Guide to Enabling a Good Death*, 2nd edn. Radcliffe, Abingdon.

Ott C, Lueger RJ, Kelber ST, Prigerson HG (2007) Spousal bereavement in older adults: common, resilient and chronic grief with defining characteristics. *Journal of Nervous and Mental Disease* 195 (4), 332–341.

Palmer E, Howarth J (2005) *Palliative Care for the Primary Care Team*. Quay Books, London.

Parkes CM (1971) The first year of bereavement: a longitudinal study of the reaction of London widows to the death of their husbands. *Psychiatry* 33, 444–467.

Parkes CM (1998) *Bereavement: Studies of Grief in Adult Life*. Penguin, London.

Parkes CM (1999) Bereavement. In: Doyle D, Hanks GWC, MacDonald N (eds) *Oxford Textbook of Palliative Medicine*, 2nd edn, pp 995–1010. Oxford University Press, Oxford.

Parkes CM, Weiss RS (1983) *Recovery from Bereavement*. Basic Books, New York.

Penson J (1990) *Bereavement: A Guide for Nurses*. Chapman and Hall, London.

Raphael B (1985) *The Anatomy of Bereavement: A Handbook for the Caring Professions*. Hutchison, London.

Raphael B (1986) *When Disaster Strikes: A Handbook for the Caring Professions*. Unwin Hyman, London.

Richards S, Hare A (1995) Issues of bereavement. In: Robbins J, Moscrop J (eds) *Caring for the Dying Patient and Family*, 3rd edn, pp 263–278. Chapman and Hall, London.

Seale C (2001) Demographic change and the experience of dying. In: Dickenson D, Johnson M, Katz JS (eds) *Death, Dying and Bereavement*, pp 35–43. Sage, London.

Steen KF (1998) A comprehensive approach to bereavement. *The Nurse Practitioner* 23 (3), 54, 59–68.

Stroebe MS, Stroebe W, Hanson RO (eds) (1993) *Handbook of Bereavement: Theory, Research and Intervention*. Cambridge University Press, Cambridge.

Stroebe M, Stroebe W, Schut H (2003) Bereavement research: methodological issues and ethical concerns. *Palliative Medicine* 17 (3), 235–240.

Stroebe W, Stroebe MS (1987) *Bereavement and Health: The Psychological and Physical Consequences of Partner Loss*. Cambridge University Press, Cambridge.

Thomas K (2003) *Caring for the Dying at Home: Companions on the Journey*. Radcliffe Medical Press, Abingdon.

Twycross R (1999) *Introducing Palliative Care*, 3rd edn. Radcliffe Medical Press, Abingdon.

Woof R, Nyatanga R (1998) Adapting to death, dying and bereavement. In: Faull C, Carter Y, Woof R (eds) *Handbook of Palliative Care*, pp 74–87. Blackwell Science, Edinburgh.

Worden JW (1991) *Grief Counselling and Grief Therapy: A Handbook for the Mental Health Practitioner*, 2nd edn. Routledge, London.

Wright B (1991) *Sudden Death: Intervention Skills for the Caring Professions*. Churchill Livingstone, Edinburgh.

Wright B (1996) *Sudden Death: A Research Base for Practice*. Churchill Livingstone, Edinburgh.

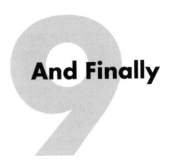

And Finally

The role of the community palliative care clinical nurse specialist is both complex and challenging. This book has given a broad overview of the work of the community palliative care clinical nurse specialist, but makes no claims to being the only interpretation of the role or, indeed, the way forward for the community palliative care clinical nurse specialist. Each individual specialist nurse will interpret and develop the role according to the needs and opportunities within her own area of clinical practice and in accordance with the needs of the local population.

For example, the role will require to be modified depending on the geographical locality within which the specialist nurse practices; the complex psychosocial and supportive needs of patients and their families living in inner city neighbourhoods may be very different from those of patients living in remote rural locations. The community palliative care clinical nurse specialist may be a sole practitioner covering a large geographical area, or part of a larger team; this will dictate, to a certain extent, her everyday workload and what she can offer to the community.

The broad framework of the clinical nurse specialist role, as described in Chapter 2, will be the foundation blocks upon which the community palliative care clinical nurse specialist develops her role and takes forward her practice. There is no doubt that the role has evolved and grown considerably over the past few years and now encompasses elements far beyond the traditional remit of direct clinical practice (Johnston 2008). The core activities of research and education are of increasing importance in today's health service and the community palliative care clinical nurse specialist is leading the way within community nursing, disseminating good practice and ensuring high quality care is available for all patients with a life-threatening illness.

The support and palliative care needs (physical, psychological, social and spiritual) of patients who are nearing the end of life, although individualised, are indeed similar and today's health and social services are working collaboratively to meet the needs of these patients. However, a number of individuals will have complex palliative care needs requiring specialist input. Caring for these individuals in the community is becoming ever more complex; patients are being nursed in their own homes with a variety of challenging nursing needs and problematic symptoms. Many of these patients who require complex nursing care or have difficult to control symptoms may have previously been nursed in the local hospital or hospice; however, they are now being given the choice to be cared for at home and to die at home.

This requires the community health and social services to deliver a service that addresses the needs of these dying patients. However, this has also resulted in the need for community health care professionals to increase their knowledge, skills and expertise in palliative care. They will be required to meet the increasingly complex medical and nursing needs of patients at home and also the supportive and emotional care of the families. The community palliative care clinical nurse specialists can meet this challenge; their commitment to personal education and development and to working collaboratively with their nursing and medical colleagues within primary care places the community palliative care clinical nurse specialist in the optimum position for taking forward palliative care in the community and providing specialist palliative care to those patients with complex care needs.

In response to the increasing demands for palliative care to take place within patients' own homes, as discussed, there will be an escalating need for education of community health care staff and social services personnel. All members of the specialist palliative care team have an ongoing commitment to education and training and to the further development of palliative care services within their own area of work. It will be incumbent on the specialist palliative care services to disseminate relevant research findings and ensure colleagues are aware of good practice. National developments such as the Gold Standards Framework (Thomas 2003) and the Liverpool Care Pathway (Ellershaw and Wilkinson 2003) are tools to assist staff in the community caring for those individuals with palliative care needs and also patients in the last days of life. These are being gradually integrated into everyday practice within the community and their positive impact on patient care will be realised with their increasing usage.

The community palliative care clinical nurse specialists have to be at the forefront of innovative practice, their role in research and education being vitally important. The community palliative care clinical nurse specialist will also be aware of the many government policies and discussion papers relating to her sphere of practice and will ensure that their proposals and recommendations are addressed and disseminated to colleagues.

Publications such as 'Cancer in Scotland: Action for Change' (Scottish Executive Health Department 2001) acknowledge the importance of palliative care and that it is not synonymous with just *terminal care*, nor is it restricted to patients with cancer, but applies to individuals with other life-threatening illnesses. A recent discussion paper from the Scottish Government, 'Better Cancer Care – A Discussion' (2008), points out that palliative care is to enable patients to achieve quality of life for the duration of their illness. It also notes the importance of the family and that the support should extend into the bereavement period. The importance of bereavement support was discussed at length in Chapter 8 of this book.

As previously mentioned, a number of these patients and their families will require specialist palliative care and access to these teams should be available to all patients with complex needs. This is, however, dependent upon referral to the service, and it is incumbent on the community palliative care clinical nurse specialist to ensure, through education, that the community health and social care professionals are aware of the role of the specialist services and in particular the role of the community palliative care clinical nurse specialist and also when referral is appropriate to the service. The National Institute for Clinical Excellence produced a paper entitled 'Improving Supportive and Palliative Care for Adults with Cancer' (2004) and acknowledged that patients with advanced cancer often experience complex problems which generalist services cannot always manage effectively and that access to specialist services should be available to all patients with complex needs.

As mentioned in Chapter 1, teamwork lies at the centre of effective palliative care. No single discipline can possibly meet all the needs and demands of dying patients and their families. It is essential that all the team members are aware of the roles of individual professionals and how and when to refer on to other services. The community palliative care clinical nurse specialist will endeavour to maintain good communication with her primary care colleagues and be readily available to discuss complex issues and make direct contact with patients and their families as requested. A large part of the role of the community palliative care clinical nurse specialist is indeed liaising with other professionals, maintaining open lines of communication and establishing and nurturing relationships with other community nurses and general practitioners. Many specialist nurses will be based in premises other than local health centres and therefore the practicalities of communication need to be addressed. The long wait outside general practitioners' offices, trying to catch them for a few minutes to discuss a patient, will be recognisable to many community nurses. The era of information technology has created an opportunity for many specialist nurses to keep in touch with both urban and rural practices and communicate more efficiently and effectively with colleagues.

The role of the community palliative care clinical nurse specialist can be very demanding, with daily exposure to death and dying; there are also difficult emotional conversations with patients and their families during most home visits. This can be painful and exhausting for even the most experienced of specialist nurses. An understanding team can do much to provide support for its members. However, the difficulties of the role can be balanced with the knowledge that the community palliative care clinical nurse specialist has the skills, knowledge and expertise to ensure that patients referred to the service with complex needs are able to die peacefully in their own home, their complex symptoms are well controlled and their families feel supported during the illness and beyond the death of the loved one into the bereavement period. The community palliative care clinical nurse specialist is not the panacea within palliative care, but merely one of the team members. It takes all the individuals within the team to deliver a service that meets the needs and demands of patients and their families. However, for many families the involvement of the community palliative care clinical nurse specialist makes a real difference.

This book has provided a very brief account of the role of the community palliative care clinical nurse specialist. It is hoped that the reader has found it informative and that it has provided a clearer understanding of the remit of the palliative care specialist nurse in the community. The author is very aware that many individuals, both professionals and the public, have limited knowledge of the work of the community palliative care clinical nurse specialist and this book has been written to try to provide a greater insight into the role. A greater appreciation of the work of the specialist nurse can be of benefit not only to patients and their families, but also to health care colleagues and all those individuals interested in palliative care who have taken time to read this book.

References

Ellershaw JE, Wilkinson S (2003) *Care of the Dying: A Pathway to Excellence*. Oxford University Press, Oxford.

Johnston G (2008) A study of a training scheme for Macmillan nurses in Northern Ireland. *Journal of Clinical Nursing* 17 (2), 242–249.

National Institute for Clinical Excellence (2004) *Improving Supportive and Palliative Care for Adults with Cancer*. National Institute for Clinical Excellence, London.

Scottish Executive Health Department (2001) *Cancer in Scotland: Action for Change*. Scottish Executive, Edinburgh.

Scottish Government (2008) *Better Cancer Care – A Discussion*. Scottish Government, Edinburgh.

Thomas K (2003) *Caring for the Dying at Home: Companions on the Journey*. Radcliffe Medical Press, Abingdon.

Index